I0430220

# Naturally I am healthy

A journey to health and well-being

Ludwig Anderson

## Disclaimer

This book is intended as an educational and informational reference.

The information provided in this book originated through personal experience and the experiences of others.

The ideas, positions and statements in this book may in some cases conflict with orthodox, mainstream medical opinion. Individual readers must assume responsibility for their own actions, safety, health, and neither the author nor the publisher shall be liable or responsible for any loss, injury, or damage allegedly arising from any information or suggestion in this book.

Note: This book might expand your view. Even though it is written by a non-native English-speaking author, it is easy to follow. As our nations grow together, it is the most beautiful thing to pass on ideas and knowledge, minimizing cultural boundaries.

# Naturally
# I am healthy

A journey to health and well-being

Ludwig Anderson

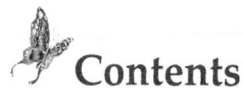 # Contents

# Preface

This little book offers a view on health, originated from life itself. It is based on the practical experience of my teachers and me.

It is intended to guide the individual to attain health and well-being.

It encourages those who are currently dealing with physical or mental disorders and looking for a permanent path to healing.

Prevention is the best medicine; therefore the contents of this book can also be seen as guidance for people wanting to live a healthy and conscious lifestyle.

Being educated to be an academic myself, I very soon had to realize the limitations of modern science. I felt there was something more significant.

It's about an intelligence or wisdom taking place on a finer and more subtle level. Too much knowledge often times obstructs pure essence.

In this era of changing consciousness, I hope to contribute to rising awareness in society and particularly to help people and animals out of chronic conditions.

Life is beautiful. You'll feel it.

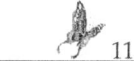

# 1. Introduction

This book is based on personal experience. It is shaped by my own search for health as well as experiences from past teachers.

How did I get to write this book?

First a few words about me.

To experience everything you are going to read now wasn't an entirely voluntary decision at the beginning. I was initially a bit shaken up, but more about this soon.

These days I'm passionate about a more natural path in life, as I 'm going to describe here. I do this with all my heart. I feel lifted. It enriches me.

I'm happier than I ever was before.

I used to be a very sick and unhappy person.

Physical suffering and mental worries made my life difficult.

By the time I finished high school I was already dealing with numerous issues concerning my health. All I wanted was to live my life, but instead, most of the time I was sitting in doctors' offices or lying in hospital beds. Starting to get chronically sick, my immune system caused me enormous trouble. The consequences were various surgeries and regular treatments with medication. I was constantly dealing with some kind of disease. So far, there was still nothing to worry about. My body was weak, but I was strong. I was young and looking forward to live my life – until I got the next slap. I contracted viral meningitis while visiting the tropics. This caused a serious brain inflammation, convulsions and neurological issues. This added upon the burden that I felt I was already carrying.

I still kept going, trying to make something out of my life.

At the age of 24, my world crashed down. I was sitting in a wheelchair.

I wasn't able to stretch my joints and muscles. My whole body was aching and burning.

I was very sick.

I started to do many different therapies and was taking strong medication.

As already mentioned, I was a young person and I had some humour left. I just thought to myself: "Here I go again. What is it this time?"

Full of confidence I gave myself to the doctors, believing in modern medicine. I was about to become an academic. Being highly convinced that 'real' scientific knowledge was the highest one could achieve, I had absolutely no doubts in modern science.

I firmly believed, "I am going to be helped."
Later I realized this was a passive approach to healing and well-being that couldn't lead me far.

There I was, lying in hospitals. Months passed and I didn't feel better. The humour I had about my disease started to disappear and the daily and nightly suffering left traces in my soul. My faith in the power of science began to rust away.
Months turned into years.
It was a nightmare.
I still thought to myself, "I will be helped" and so I went from one therapy to another. I sought help at modern doctors and physical therapists.
Luckily I couldn't have asked for better doctors. They were competent and honest. I got the best treatments in the most advanced and specialised clinics western medicine can imagine. People deeply cared for me and wanted to help me relieve my symptoms.
Many treatments gave me some relief in my suffering, but they couldn't resolve them.
I still felt bad and side effects of the medication began to show up.
I was dealing with strong pain all over my body and often-times I suffered from fever.
I felt very sick and couldn't sleep.

More and more complications and pain piled up.

I had become a wreck.

I was only able to endure my situation while being on severe drugs prescribed by my doctors. I thought to myself, "I will live a few years shorter now, but at least I'll get some life. That's still better than not living at all!"

What a shame to this beautiful gift of life, but back then the situation seemed to be more than hopeless to me.

In a more or less gentle way specialists tried to let me know that I would be disabled for the rest of my life and that it would do me better to accept the situation as it is. It would be necessary to adjust my life and dreams according to it. I was devastated.

Nevertheless, I was dependent on the medical system. I was grateful for having support and for having strong medication available that made my life kind of manageable.

Yet, I was constantly dealing with severe pain and new diseases started to show up, which often-times required hospitalisation. What kind of a life was that?

Years passed and I started to realize that if things were going to continue like this, I would be dead soon. I felt very desperate. I had tried the best I could. I had done everything to get well. I didn't have any hope left. All I did was try to make it through the day – and through the night.

It's a fact; everything that is alive is also subject to change.

I was no exception.

I packed an entire piece of luggage with prescribed medication and went away. I did this several times. Of course, each time I did that, I ended up being hospitalised abroad. For every country I have been to, I know exactly what the hospitals look like.

Different people started to show up in my life.

At the height of this vicious circle, many years of suffering had passed. I was 31 years old and took a minimum of 1500 different prescription pills per year. I didn't want to take all these and kept the dose as low as I could. I had already taken a total of roughly 10,000 tablets of various medications in the past seven years.

It was time to make a change if I still wanted to get out of this alive.

Fortunately, I met people who had a good influence on me and gave me lots of inspiration. They led me to a relevant path of healing.

At the beginning I wasn't receptive to that. I was convinced of the supremacy of modern science and whenever I had tried a more natural approach, it had always felt inappropriate, suitable for 'housewives' and diseases like a light cough. I was stubborn and arrogant.

Over the years incredible people started to show up into my life. These people began to show me alternative ways of living.

I was observing healthy, shining people, full of life and joy, having strong bodies and happy faces. I could witness many of the ways in which they lived, for example eating flowers and doing yoga every morning at 6am.

"Come on now… eating flowers?!"

I wasn't taking them for serious at all.

"Dreamers", I thought.

The way they lived, the things they did, were like peanuts to me: nice, even a bit crazy, but definitely not my thing. I wasn't convinced. I didn't see any relation to my life and my chronic condition. Yet, subconsciously, I guess I might have gotten a little bit influenced.

A few years later I met a yoga teacher. He was in his seventies. I observed him for a while. He looked so alive. His physical abilities and his kind personality made me curious.

"He must have always been well", I thought.

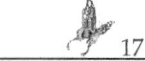 

"Lucky him, he probably did all of this his entire lifetime."

I wanted to show him my respect and went over to talk to him.

"No", he said.

"When I was 58, I was walking with a stick. I had so much pain in my body that I thought my life was over."

"But how is this possible", I asked him, already feeling that something important was about to happen.

"Oh, I changed my lifestyle", he said.

"I will tell you what to do and where to get more information".

This meeting lasted only five minutes, but it was about to change my entire life. That was the time when I finally got familiar with the health education of the free minded author *Franz Konz*, a cancer survivor, health advocate author. A large part of this book is inspired by his life's work.

These days I am deeply in love with my life. I am enjoying each single moment. I found happiness and well-being. I feel strong and the only time I am entering a hospital is when I am visiting others.

The lifestyle I am about to describe here had a radical positive impact on me. Additionally, thousands of

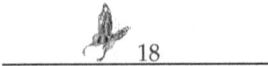 

other people have improved their lives via the inspired teachings of Franz Konz and other pioneers like him.

Let us now ask the following questions:
How can one achieve permanent well-being or even a cure?
What needs to be considered and implemented to get on that relevant path of healing?
Take heart. It's possible and it's for free. You don't need anyone and you're completely independent.
You'll feel fantastic and a high quality of life is waiting for you.

# 2. Preparation

What should you begin with in order to be naturally healthy?

First, it is important to look at yourself and your suffering. Take it seriously. Don't take your illness and your life superficially. Instead look closely at it.

Don't fall into self-pity either and don't whine to everyone. It is now time for you to actively take over your recovery.

In order to do that, you have to take yourself and your needs seriously, especially in front of yourself. If you don't take yourself seriously and if you don't accept yourself, how then should other people take you seriously and accept you?

Be more important to yourself, especially if you're very ill. Your health has priority now. It's time to start actively taking care of you.

Make a clear decision and stick to it.

Open your eyes and look at yourself.

How do you live and how are you?

Do you really want your life continuing like this?

Do you want to continue sobbing, waiting for a miracle to happen?

Look at it closely.

Isn't it finally time to give your body and soul what they really need?

Maybe you're currently not sure how to accomplish this. Something else has always been more important, or perhaps someone else?
The inner attitude towards oneself is an important attitude for healing. Taking yourself seriously will convert more and more into self-love. This love will then spread to other people, animals and plants.

You will also need some patience.
We would like to override natural time sequences, but natural timing is as it is.
It is precise.
Often-times we want solutions as quickly as possible. We want to transform natural time sequences according to our wishes. Mostly we would like to speed things up. On the other hand, some things we would like to slow down, like our aging process to name an example.
We want everything to work exactly in time as it pleases our will to happen. If it doesn't, then we still try to make it happen, until it does, even if it is by force. Then we use violence to our bodies and our souls. Despite discomfort, we stuff them with fast

pills to operate and drive in the fast lane, instead of giving natural processes and procedures time and space.

"But, but ...." The words are screaming there within you.

"I need that."

"I can't, I have to ..."

Think about the fact, that if you're keeping this up, you might not be able to do anything. Always make sure to take good care of yourself.

What exactly will happen if you decide to give yourself and everything around you a little bit more time?

Think.

Breathe.

What will happen if you should start to follow your body's and soul's signals?

What exactly are you afraid of? Are you afraid of less income? Do you feel fear of losing friends or disappointing your family by having less time? You will miss something "important"?

I am asking you now, what are your priorities?

Of course, the day has only 24 hours. Consider well how you spend them.

In the end, it might not just be you taking benefit, but also your professional life and fellow human beings.

Do you really think you're going to starve by giving yourself and things in your life a bit more time? Sometimes less can be more.

But no, you can't.
You have to. You have to….
"But…."
"And anyway…."
"…an absurdity such a thing!"

Maybe you'll have to let go a little. You might even feel it's a good thing to do.
Maybe you'll instead gain something new, something that might enrich you even more. Instead, something better might come into your life, something you don't know yet, something that currently seems to be out of reach.
If you want to implement something new, you need to create space first, meaning you have to remove things or concepts. Where else could new things take place?
If you're really sick, you will probably have no choice anyway. You already hit rock bottom and have nothing to lose, right?
Most things take time.
Look how long it takes until an apple is ripe.

First the tree has to grow and prosper. Then flowers are pollinated. Nevertheless, many months have to pass until slowly and deliberately the tree bears fruit. After all this time of nurturing, imagine how delicious and juicy these fruits taste. They are full of life force.

Our body is nothing more than another organism, perfectly equipped by creation. Trust that your system[1] is able to bring itself back into balance, provided you give it the opportunity to do so!

Take a look at all the processes in your body. What happens if you cut yourself and bleed or if you've swallowed something down the wrong way? Think about all the processes your system automatically performs day and night. It is inhaling and digesting. It is constantly creating new cells. You cannot be serious thinking our body is not intelligent! Do we really have to interfere, thinking we know better?

Our system follows certain laws, mercilessly adhering to them. Everything is made in a perfect way. Realize these laws are not made by us, but only

---

[1] In this book the word 'system' shall describe the human organism as a dynamic and complex interconnection between body, soul, mind and spirit.

by nature. You are a marvel of nature. Therefore stop disturbing your body in its quest for balance. Instead live more according to nature's laws.

Unfortunately these ways are not always what we want.

Illness and suffering are indicating that there's something about your life your system doesn't like at all. There's something about the way you live bringing your body out of its natural balance. It can no longer function with the lifestyle you're providing. It tries to work things out, doing its best by compensating the unbalance. It also starts to send automatic warning signals, "Attention, attention, if you keep this up, our survival is threatened."

Feelings of discomfort are nothing to fight with, but are early messages of your body, like notes from a friend.

Listen up. Do not overlook it. It's your life.

Even if you don't listen, keeping things up as before, your body follows natural laws, being its guidance.

It responds to your lifestyle.

If you sit a lot, you'll get back pain. If you're eating too many candies, you might get cavities. Drinking too much alcohol, you might throw up.

Many bodily symptoms are easy to understand. At the beginning your system always tries to get rid of things, things that don't belong in it. Eventually the cost might get too high. You wouldn't survive constantly throwing up. In order to survive, our system finds other solutions.

So-called diseases are primarily rescue attempts of your body. They are healing and clean-up processes.

Remember, your body is very smart!

What happens if you're tired? Your body or mind might need some rest, perhaps in order to process or simply to restore.

What's wrong with that? You're not a machine, even though you are surrounded by many.


Maybe you've never listened to your body and you have let it degenerate.

Maybe you didn't know any better. If that's the case, then it is likely you might get some diseases, which I don't wish upon you.

You don't want to live in a garbage dump, right? Your life energy doesn't like to live in a garbage dump either.

We complain about all these bad viruses and all those nasty bacteria, but in nature, which we are only a part of, even those have an important function: decomposing things that are no longer viable, which no longer work.

Natural medicine has a well-known saying, "There are no bad bacteria and viruses; it's the breeding ground that matters."

Take care and create a healthy environment within your system. You'll have less unwanted guests, as there is going to be less to decompose. I know it sounds harsh, but in nature there are no reviews. Things are completely unbiased. They are as they are.

If you're not healthy or happy by living your current lifestyle, what could you change and how?

Do you want to change anything?

How exactly would a lifestyle look approximating nature's laws?

How can the body and soul work in harmony again, finding their way back to a beautiful union of health?

How can all your cells perform their very own functionality, firm and perfectly programmed by nature?

It is possible to reach well-being again. Our lifestyle needs to change by living in a way that has been intended and programmed for us.

My teacher, Franz Konz, always used to say, "There are no diseases, but only wrong ways of living."

Very soon in this book, we'll get to the part of how we can implement this idea accurately, even in society.

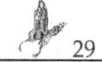

# 3. We are our nature

Our present age is strongly influenced by theories and technology. Nevertheless, we are alive, just like everything else in nature is alive.

Where do you actually classify yourself on our planet?

Don't forget that you're not one of these machines you're surrounded with on a daily basis. You are alive and thus a natural part of the ecosystem.

Step outside and take a closer look at nature now. Each time you will see something natural. Put your awareness on what is surrounding you. Don't just walk by. Don't just pass, entangled in thoughts. Try to be open. Observe plants, trees, shrubs, flowers and weeds of your area. You might even see some animals here and there.

It is so amazing seeing everything engages together in a perfectly adapted ecosystem. Isn't it a marvel that brings one to wonder?

Every organism has its purpose in life that it's destined to perform quite naturally, without any complaint or stepping out of line assuming humans don't interfere in nature's system.

Everything is perfect.

Let's take a simple example.

A bee is flying from flower to flower because it feeds on it. This also matches the intentions of the plant. The flowers' bright red or yellow colours can be seen as signals, "Hello, here I am. Come to me."

The bee automatically takes care of the flower too, because through the continuous transfer of pollen it contributes to its pollination and thus it secures the species' existence. This can happen in several ways. Some plants grow fruits, which in turn have attractive colours so that other animals, such as birds or mammals get attracted to them. They eat the ripe fruits and excrete the seeds. They contribute to the plant's propagation elsewhere.

Everyone takes benefit. The plants profit, the animals are well fed and move on their way.

In creation, everyone and everything has its place.

I am asking you again: Where is our place?

It's amazing. Even the smallest creature has its meaning and purpose.

Let's take ants as an example. Sometimes we might feel them to be so annoying.

It's great to watch them.

What are they actually doing?

Try to observe them for a while. You might realize how clean they are, how they tidy up.

They cut and carry away everything that is dead and broken.

There are even trees living in symbiosis with ants. They keep the tree and its whole environment clean, warding off intruders too. In return the tree provides them with habitat and food.

Just go outside and take a closer look. Every day you will recognize something new. You may enjoy it! Creation is full of harmony, symbiosis and perfection.

We're just another part of it, even if we might have forgotten.

Why should it be different with us?

Nature follows complex rules.

It acts according to its very own laws. Nothing and no one can change that, including us.

Creation is perfect and takes care of all its organisms. It's strong.

The very nature of laws made every life arise and these laws are certainly not created by humans.

Being in our comfort zone, we thought we could master nature. We wanted to dominate and exploit it. We are important, yes, but we are just as important as a beetle or an ant. Nature makes no difference in treating their creatures.

Everything is part of creation, having its meaning and purpose.

Yes, your importance to the planet is the same as a beetle or an ant. Regarding our current lifestyle, I'd say that they're even more important than us, because at least they stick to their assigned life. They don't destroy the planet, unlike us humans. Humans are the only organisms that think it's possible to step out of line.

Go into nature.

You'll find yourself very small. Yet you're connected to it. You are nature.


Even though we're treating creation quite badly, it continues to provide us with energy, sun, water and light, meaning food and warmth. If we could only leave it this way! It is full of love and has so much to give.

It might not fit your wishful thinking, but one thing is certain:

Nothing, absolutely nothing, can rise above it.

We try to invent a thousand things, but in the end they cause us even more problems. Unfortunately, we mainly realize this later. Why don't we just live in harmony, according to creation's laws like all other living beings in the first place?

Nature could exhale deeply, just once, and we are all gone!

So-called natural disasters in particular can be quite simply seen as an example of how small and powerless we are. One deep exhalation, be it a storm, an earthquake or a meteorite impact – do you really think that's exhausting for nature?

I don't think so.

If creation decides so, life on this planet and even in space can end each moment and you're completely powerless against it.

Finally, become humble and stick to creations' laws. It is wiser and more intelligent than any human being on this planet can ever be. It is the author of nature's laws, having everything perfectly designed, so that things can work.

The validity of its laws will not change. They are authentic and invariable, in contrast to people's insights, which change from century to century or even from year to year. Yet we're repeatedly taken in by so-called scholars and think:

"Yes, now they have figured it out. The mystery is revealed!"

Things that are currently declared to be right, should then be valid for everyone until – yes, until eventually they turn out to be wrong. Something new has been found valid and everyone is nodding in full agreement without having even inspected what is really going on, applying a clear mind and heart.

If you really think about it, doesn't it appear a bit weird to you too?

We will never be able to be more important or to be wiser and larger than forces and laws of nature and creation. Realize, surrender and practice yourself in awe.

Attempting to penetrate creation's mysteries, particularly trying to control it, is a figment of stray people living too much in their mind.

Stick to the rules and live in harmony with nature, like all other organisms do.

You are no exception.

Read it again closely: You are no exception.

Why should you be one?

Leave your old perspective behind, to be something special in creation, to have a special position in it.

What do we really know?

Is our medical system really able to heal chronically sick individuals and make them healthy?

Do you still believe a miracle will happen?

So much money is being dissipated in research and science, but in the end it doesn't change anything.

People still suffer from rheumatism. They die of cancer and get a dozen heart attacks. Diagnoses like 'irritable bowel syndrome' are made. What for?

Nothing has changed, except for a shift of suffering and a more pleasant decoration in the doctoring up of statistics.

It won't change anything. There are always going to be new things needing to be 'fought'. Hasn't this always been the case?

Approaching life like this, nothing will change. We need to follow a completely different path. We must turn from this one way street being sold to us as a motorway.

Once again, in this creation you don't have any exceptional function.


Do you think everything you see and hear is all that exists?

There are even animals, yes, these 'lower' creatures are able to see, hear and sense much more than you do.

They can hear sounds and see things that we don't perceive with our senses.

There is always more existing around us, even if we can't grasp it.

What kind of eyes do we have?

One of these days you should go out at night into nature, all by yourself, without a flashlight.
Try it once in practice, because then you'll see how powerful we really are.

When I roam through the countryside, I get some interesting thoughts sometimes.
Once, I was in the woods, collecting plants.
I looked on the forest floor and saw a beetle running around in the forest probably unspeakably large for him.
"How interesting", I thought.
"Perhaps we are also like this beetle here. It has certainly never seen a car or people. It knows nothing and assumes that what it perceives is the only thing that exists."
Perhaps we are also like a beetle and scurry around in our own little world, firmly believing there's only that. Perhaps we're also too small to perceive anything beyond on any sensory level whatsoever.
What do we really know?
Do we really claim to understand existence between heaven, earth and beyond?
We know nothing.
It is impossible to perceive what else exists around us or better said what could exist around us.

In the end it's about realizing that we're living beings firmly embedded in nature's large ecosystem. In creation's sense and favour, we're subjected to its laws and rules like all other organisms on this planet. Turning our lives away from nature's laws doesn't just bring damage to our planet and all its living beings in an irresponsible way; no, it also brings damage to you personally; it brings you suffering and disease.

Let us therefore listen to creation's laws and simply live by them.

Let us finally take some steps forward.

Let's approach a lifestyle matching creation a bit more, leading us to our place in it.

# 4. A species appropriate way of life

We are now getting to the core of this book.

In the following we will find answers to the questions of how to approach a species appropriate way of life in a practical way.

It is about attaining well-being and clarity, about being happy. We will discuss a lifestyle according to the applicable laws of nature in the modern world.

The idea of living a natural lifestyle is nothing new. A variety of information of how to approach this path can be found in abundance. General advice on health has always been available, as attaining health and well-being has been of great importance to most people. Some of this advice is of great value, and therefore, recommendable.

So many different opinions can be found when it comes to food. Modern people have even started to welcome a more vegetarian or raw type of diet. Talking about edible plants is also getting more common.

Experts highly recommend to move our bodies a lot, to exercise sufficiently. Diverse exercise programs are being offered in order to take care of our health, be it yoga, Nordic walking, visiting a gym, etc.

On the soul level, we can find numerous approaches, not fitting into one single book. You can learn different relaxation techniques, get consultation or select esoteric approaches.

All of these programs are useful and you certainly can benefit by applying them into your life. In my opinion, we are mostly lacking a holistic approach on all levels, being part of everyday life and not just a therapy session along the way. The desired goal of long-term health and balance is therefore seldom achieved. The individual remains searching, feeling unfulfilled.

We are highly complex organisms, perfectly matched. One thing interlocks with the other, as it is in all of nature. We are only a small part of it and yet completely embedded therein. One thing works only with the other. In order to achieve real health and well-being, all levels – diet, exercise, soul and habitat – are supposed to be brought together into balance. Our health depends on all these levels and each level in turn depends on all other levels.

Below I will talk about these aforementioned levels.

If you want to use this information, integrate all four levels into your life, not just one of them.

I am now going to explain one of these four levels.

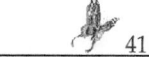 

As already mentioned, this part is only complete with all the other layers being described later on.

# I. Species appropriate nutrition

Imagine all creatures come into this world and everything they need is already here. Everything is perfectly created. Each organism knows what to eat and where to find food. They know where to sleep and how to ensure their species' survival. It is amply provided for them.

Human culture hasn't been here for a very long time. Compare it to our planet's existence and to the existence of flora and fauna.

Human beings, however, got obsessed, having the idea of taking a special role in creation. Believing man is something special, has been enforced through power, religion and fear, carried on over generations.

Creation cares for all living beings equally, provided they live according to its laws. Imagine also you would get into this world and everything is already here.

Just try to imagine.

Except us, every organism on this planet can live without any inventions, just the way they are.

They remain in natural interconnection, following their inner rhythm.

Why are we the only organism incapable of doing this?

Should life be really determined for us this way?

Are we not also loved by creation, born into a world that provides for us?

Let's have a look at our closest relatives, the great apes.

In biological systematics humans are mammals of the 'primates' class. The great apes are referred to as primates on the same level just like us, classifying them in the same family. Among the great apes family are included chimpanzees, bonobos, gorillas and humans. This classification on the same level was introduced a few decades ago because genetic comparisons couldn't deny similarities any longer. Earlier, human beings were placed in a separate family.

This idea, however, has become out-dated. It has lost validity.

These days we officially belong to one family, along with the great apes.


How do our relatives feed themselves in the wild?

How do we feed oursleves in comparison?

Why is it that our closest relatives eat so differently than we do?

They even feel good with it. They love, laugh and frolic, having an incredible fitness.

I'm not talking about those poor creatures, doomed to be locked up in the zoo, getting their meals prescribed by humans. I'm talking about the few survivors still being found in their natural habitat.

Why should our diet differ so much from theirs?

Let us leave this question open for now.

Let's go back to imagining that nature is perfect, that everything is provided for us.

Does it also provide us with cooking pots, pans, blenders, microwaves, ovens and large factories?

Can you find this in nature?

How long have nature's laws already reigned?

How long has human civilization been in existence?

Try to compare these dimensions and then start to marvel. Ask yourself where truth and essence really can be found.

Human beings and their genetic constitution are certainly subject to evolution. They are adapting and changing.

That's probably true and who knows what human beings will become in 500,000 years.

Evolutionary changes don't happen as quickly as we think they do, however. There are temporal gaps between rapid technological changes and the spread of civilization on one side and the actual adaption of human's organisms on the other side. It's just the way. In body and soul there's still the same original program dwelling, given to us by nature a long time ago as the perfect solution for a harmonious life here on this planet, including all its inhabitants. Everything should already be perfect for us.

Unfortunately, we developed a different view, losing confidence in our home, which is nature.

We are building an alternative world, a civilization. Actually, we already know all this. The contrast of current lifestyle to original programming made us name many diseases. We are talking about so-called 'diseases of civilization'.

Thus we're already aware of our lifestyle not contributing to long-term health, nor to our planet's health.

Something must be wrong.

Nevertheless, we don't really change anything about it.


If our organism would be really adjusted to our current way of life, we would have an oversized head and be more flexed in the hips, as we mainly sit as much as possible, using our brain more than the rest of our body.

We still have an upright posture (at least that's the normal case) and our limbs, particularly the legs, make up the largest part of our body's proportion.

It's a fact that we currently possess this appearance. This has very specific causes, and of course, consequences as well.

What does all of this have to do with our diet?
If we take a look around in nature, we can see that all living beings, without exception, eat what they can find in nature. They eat the food that is intended for them, unless human beings interfere. If man doesn't interfere, everyone and everything lives according to their very own programming, in harmony and union with creation. Animals roam, eating leaves, roots and fruits or other living creatures. Predators hunt and eat fresh meat, caught without any tools and extra help, but with their own body features. They are perfectly made for this task and function.

Due to its own program and design, every living being is exactly made for a certain lifestyle and a certain habitat. Normally it lives entirely consistent in a matched manner, whether it's the snake, the fish or the spider.

The great apes, primates like us, have arms, legs, hands and feet. Our relatives roam on the ground and climb in trees. Food consists of things they can get with their own body features, living in an environment where they can always find food.

What exactly do they eat?

They don't cook. They don't hunt large animals.

What do they actually live on, especially being so incredibly agile and strong?

In general, food is made of leaves, fruits, berries, roots, bark, seeds, nuts, insects and micro-organisms. These are things they can find in their natural habitat. They find it on their own without much effort.

Creation is so smart and generous.


Let's take a look at us human beings. We have already heard about similarities to our closest relatives. We can become less vain to make this kind of approach. The similarities are too big to deny or do you still think you're something better?

Let's take a look at our physical attributes and our musculoskeletal system. Our posture is very upright. Our legs are straight, longer than our arms. Thus, it is undeniable that we are made to walk and run. Why else would those legs have been given to us? Permanent sitting was certainly not part of the programming.

Our bodies can also bend down or crawl, yet it's not comparable to a cow's physique.

Envision a cow's image.

Is its physique determined to climb trees or isn't it rather perfectly equipped to eat grass all day long, due to its posture?

We humans have two agile arms and fine motor finger skills.

We would also be much fitter and more skilful; more than we can ever imagine if we would only had continued to stay in motion. We would be very fit if we needed to rely on it. Our organism's potential is huge. Remember all these physical performances certain people, mostly athletes, are capable of.

This body equipment was given to us by creation.

Do you really want to overlook this part of your life, just as if it wouldn't exist?

All of this has to make some kind of sense somehow! Nature is perfectly programmed. Don't forget that.


Nobody really likes to hear this, but it is as it is. Human beings should walk, run, roam, climb, stoop, stretch, reach out and thus take food from nature.

We should eat this food as it is found, without subjecting it to inventions, without any changing processes.

All living beings do well behaving naturally, as it is designed for their system.

We should also try to approach that kind of lifestyle.

Everything you are going to read here might sound weird at the very beginning, and probably like something your mind needs to get used to.

I certainly don't mean to say that from now on you should climb naked in the trees all day long, searching for food, although you 're welcome to try, if you want to do something funny.

It is more about getting a deep understanding. It is about your proper place in this world and the consequences for your life. This part of the book is about a diet that makes you healthy again, that reconciles you with your programming and thus helps you to be happy and satisfied.

Let's look at the whole thing a little more closely.

We human beings can walk a lot, and while doing this, we can bend and squat down to eat herbs, flowers and other plants from the ground, including leaves and berries of shrubs. We can stretch, reach out, jump and throw. Thus, we can also eat leaves and fruits of larger shrubs and trees. Finally we can eat even more by climbing up the trees. Due to our complex body functions, our ability to move around and our fine motor skills, a variety of pure food and life forces becomes available to us. They might even be intended for us.

Man can also run.

We would have to if we'd live in nature in order to quickly find a safe place, like climbing up a tree.

Are we really fast enough and are we able to regularly kill an animal on our own power or to catch a big fish from the sea without weapons and other support devices? I think on a regular long term basis this would be very difficult. Then the prey, of course, needs to be eaten just like that: raw. Whether it is possible or not, transforming your life shouldn't fail due to this detail.

If you're currently eating meat and fish, then check one thing: How does it feel to you, going into the real practice of your food's origin?

To be exact, look for someone like a hunter or a fisherman and accompany him. Ask him to help you as much as necessary to hunt the prey on your own. Kill it yourself if you can. Prepare it with his help. This is a bloody affair.

If you can't eat the whole thing raw, then cook it and eat it right away. Only then you can really make a decision and not live in unconsciousness any longer. You will then know what your eating is really about.

These days, our main supply of fish and meat looks quite differently. It has become more of a factory production rather than 'just' a hunting process.

Helping in a slaughterhouse for just a few hours would actually be a better way to open up our awareness. These institutions usually don't let you enter.

Therefore, friends of mine went to a biological slaughterhouse and got a 'tour'. After that, their meat consumption changed immensely. Even what they saw on a sustainably managed slaughterhouse troubled them deeply.

I think it's very important, especially for young people, to get opportunities to be able to make a conscious decision, having a real reference to their food's origin.

Young people get thrown and pressured into society so cluelessly. What's the big deal about installing an excursion to a slaughterhouse in high school? Everyone is eating meat, so where is the problem? There shouldn't be anything bad about taking a closer look...


Let's back up now and talk about species appropriate nutrition.

Living in nature would be like eating what is right around us, resources of food we're able to reach easily.

Why should it be made difficult for us?

Everything is already there. It's simple and easy.

Why should we not ingest leaves, herbs, seeds, flowers, bark, fruits, berries, roots and micro-organisms such as insects?

We should do this in pure form, meaning to eat everything as it is found, without any altering process. We should stop believing that we have a special role on this planet.

Could all this really be possible? You should eat the leaves of trees?

Yes, even I had to laugh about all that in the beginning.

Now, I've been doing this for years. It is not only remained with me, but even friends and family got into wild plants. This kind of nutrition agrees with me splendidly, especially after overcoming initial inhibitions and some small taste adaptations. I didn't encounter a single problem and others did not complain either.

For anyone having doubts, it really is extremely compatible. On the contrary, the body and soul begin to shine and to be happy. Finally they get what they need, what is intended for them.

You'll be amazed at how well it feeds you. After a transition period of a few months, you'll start to build a beautiful, slim, strong body.

Don't be afraid and have faith in creation. However, stick to its rules.

Ingredients found in wild plants have immense value.

Unfortunately, with wild plants there's little monetary gain to be made. Only few studies have been made, but even those have shown how powerful wild plants are and that a high amount of protein can be found in green leaves.

Why do you imagine a gorilla is that big and strong, even though it's mainly eating leaves the whole day?

Where do its muscles come from?

Where does it get all its powers from?

It doesn't even eat fish or meat.

I know, at the beginning all of this is hard to believe.

We already have departed so far from our origin, which is nature.

From now on be more natural and you'll start to shine very strongly from the inside and the outside.

How about milk and cheese?

No matter what kind of question may get into your mind, this is just one example. From now on you can find answers to your own question. You could also think about bread or soup.

Always ask yourself: Is it natural?

Is it available for me as a human in nature without using massive tools, or is it not?

Try to imagine yourself in the wild, running behind a non-domesticated cow, trying to get something out of its udder. It is likely you'll get a quick response from the cow.

A cow's milk is intended for its own calves. Only for that purpose it was established by creation and certainly not for feeding us.

Imagine all the things humans prepare from milk.

From now on, it is about seeing more clearly.

What are we eating throughout the day?

Check out your breakfast tomorrow.

What are you having for lunch?

How does dinner look?

How much of pure nature are you currently taking into you?

What would your food look like if you'd pay more attention to your natural programming?

If you take a look at society, at eating patterns that we have arranged out of pleasure and comfort, you would be shocked.

How much we depend on it! There's a real defence when it comes to food, especially regarding associated taste experiences.

Who is the master in your house?

Do you really have to be a slave of your desires, involuntarily being at its mercy?
Should you and your programming not instead decide what you're taking into your system, rather than being dictated by society and desires?
Become free.

Do you think you're already eating quite healthy according to conventional standards?
The choice of words is also important. We shouldn't eat, but nourish ourselves. Even using a different word, 'nourish' instead of 'eating' is quite significant. Do you make sure to always buy whole grains? Do you eat plenty of fruits and vegetables, cook with natural ingredients and indulge yourself only now and then in a piece of chocolate, maybe two?
Unfortunately, there is a lack of education on this subject. People mostly stopped thinking on their own and blindly follow what others, mainly scientists and industrialists, make them believe. In society it is common to willingly work with the most powerful means of persuasion in humanity: fear.
Free yourself. Begin to think on your own. Start to decide for yourself.
Don't be afraid. Be courageous and be alive.
Natural food is not only meant for you.

It goes beyond that. It is going to renew you and stream through you from head to toe, because it is pure life energy and vitality.

It arises directly from our planet Earth, with all its nutrients. At the same time it got nurtured with pure life energy from our sun.

Natural, fresh food contains so many minerals, vitamins, enzymes, chlorophyll and other life substances of which we know nothing.

All this takes place in a unique organic compound, a unique composition that can never be imitated by any human being.

Taking fresh wild food within you, you'll be a part of everything. Your health and your well-being are going to increase immensely.

Eat this food as it is: raw and unwashed. Don't subject it to any kind of process. Everything is meant for you, exactly as it is. Bees and bugs might have visited the plant before you did and maybe they have left some pollen or soil particles here and there. There are also other things being left on the plant. You just can't see them with your eyes.

Micro-organisms and their excretions, pollen and the remains of soil are important food components you automatically take into your system while eating, creating an excellent base for your intestinal flora.

After a while, you will be stunned at how strong your immune system has become and how all your regular ailments just disappear.

I wish more research would be done on wild plants' ingredients, on green leaves in general, so that more people can get access to this issue and trust in it.


Let's talk about cooking, about general food preparation.

Nature provides no cooking pots and pans for their creatures. Have you ever seen an animal cooking?

It's an invention of man, a very recent one.

What was going on with our mind when we started all that?

Why should we take such a special position in nature?

If you cook something, you're changing it. It is then something different compared to what it used to be, even if it's a natural product. By cooking a raw potato, you turn an incompatible food to a compatible feed.

Through the cooking process, you therefore change its properties. It is a different product as a result.

By cooking, you may turn poisonous plants to something edible. However, it is questionable whether this kind of plant originally was intended for you. Maybe it was meant to be for another living creature on this planet.

When cooking food, it is most important to keep in mind that almost all valuable ingredients get destroyed. They are important building materials of life previously mentioned: vitamins, enzymes, chlorophyll, micro-organisms, and life energy.

Of course, cooked food also provides energy, which can be used and burned, but what an effort for our system to exploit this and what type of energy is it?

It is lacking any important life substances. It is sort of a lifeless energy.

Imagine I throw you into the saucepan. What will happen then? You'll be thrown into it alive and in a few seconds you're dead.

You die, just like your food.

Next time you're going to have a meal, take a look at your filled plate.

What does your food actually look like? Does it look limp, hanging and mushy from all the cooking? Do you have to chew at all?

What are we doing to our food?

Yes, it tastes good.

Is this habitual taste more important to you than health and happiness? Is an enjoyment of minutes on

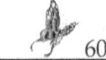

your taste buds more important to you than 24 hours full of well-being and happiness?

If this is really the case, it's up to you to decide to go for it. Make your choice in full awareness, but also stop complaining if you might feel bad.

In terms of a modern diet, it's not just the cooking process, harming us the most.

Invented substances, chemical additives, which these days can be found in our food, are even more threatening to our system. In addition we are facing new dangers:

Genetically engineered foods, commonly known as gmo, are already spreading at breakneck speed.

My teacher Franz Konz used to say, "These things are not for us. It is like going to a strange planet in order to eat stones from there. Our body has absolutely no idea what to do with them. Our system isn't familiar with all these substances. They don't belong to it. It is not our program."

What should your system do with all these things? How should it handle something that was never intended for it? What to do with all these chemicals we're absorbing with every meal we take, all the drugs we need?

Chemicals are the greatest harm to your health.

Avoid them as much as you can. They put you out of balance, disturb your system's innate intelligence, gradually increasing more confusion until eventually it's too late.

Step over to your kitchen now and take a look at your food's ingredients, food that you really like, that you eat on a daily basis. In some cases this might not be possible. Just take bread as an example. Even if you go to get it at a bakery, 'fresh and homemade', you would be surprised to find out about its ingredients.

Just go and check your products. I'll wait.

By reading the packaging, you now have taken a closer look at your food's ingredients.

Doesn't all this give you a better understanding of what you're actually doing to yourself? It's almost impossible to really understand what the chemicals are you're getting to read on the packaging.

We might therefore end up thinking, "So what? What I don't know won't hurt me."

What you get to read about your products and their ingredients really doesn't seem that bad, but what do they actually mean?

Do you understand what is written on your products, ingredients you are daily taking to you?

Do you really know exactly what is hiding behind all the cleverly camouflaged terms?

Don't let yourself be fooled by all the producers and manufacturers. It's all about money. Everyone wants to have it, isn't that the case?

For them, the point is to acquire profit and not taking care of their custumors' personal health.

Everything is so appealing. Everything is packaged nicely. There can't be anything bad inside.

The product's outside might show pictures of smiling families, happy children or be marked '100% natural' and 'no additives'. After seeing this you can't help but buy it.


Imagine, in a cup of fruit yogurt about eight cubes of sugar are hidden. A big container of pickled red cabbage contains about 25 sugar cubes and the portion of cornflakes in the morning gives you a 12 sugar cubes dose. A can of pineapple can contain up to 18 sugar cubes and a small glass of champagne flips you directly with two cubes of sugar in your system.

One can hardly imagine what is really contained in our food. Is it any wonder we are suffering from so many, often new diseases?

Wake up and think on your own.

Think of what you're doing in an autopilot mode every single day. Don't be a robot. Don't let yourself be blindly carried away by everything that surrounds you.

Imagine where all these attractively packaged products come from. They probably originate in one of those many big grey food-industrial-cooperate-factory apparatuses where your products' ingredients are merged with chemicals into huge boilers, processed by many machines, by many different hands. Then, the whole thing goes over many assembly lines and through more equipment until it is finally ready in your grocery store. Of course it is all nicely packaged by then.

If you're unlucky, you might get an additional panic attack while waiting in line at the constantly beeping supermarket checkout.


I prefer to go outside instead. Being surrounded by peace and quiet, I look for some dandelion and maybe pluck a juicy apple, both shining with full life power, while listening to chirping birds.

I could also go to an organic farmer and carefully choose nice lettuce, some herbs and fresh fruit. I might even talk to the farmer like a human being.

How much have we disconnected from our nature?

Turn away from chemicals and processed food.

Instead, choose the purity and freshness of living nature.

You are what you eat, so it is often said.

You'll feel that you become more and more alive, just like your food.

Deep satisfaction and mental clarity will reward you. Wild plants have a high nutritional value, including very common weed plants. Don't be too proud to eat something like that. Don't be too comfortable for it either. It's really simple. Uncomfortable is actually just changing your habits and the rest will happen by itself.

Of course you'll need to learn a little bit about a plant's edibility before starting, but more about that in chapter six.

For now keep in mind to eat your food as fresh, unchanged and natural as possible. You can choose from all kinds of edible plants. You can eat many different leaves or flowers. There are a variety of edible fruits and berries with great taste. Seeds, nuts and roots are also nourishing. All of this you can find almost anywhere. You can just go outside and serve yourself.

I often do not have the time or abilities to go foraging myself, in which case I go shopping.

I didn't mean to say you should immediately pack your backpack, leaving everything and everyone behind.

All of this is about getting an understanding of how it might be at its optimum. If you understand this, you can then try to imitate species appropriate nutrition, adapted to your current living conditions.

Of course, you can also feed just from nature if you dispose of the necessary environment and have enough discipline to do it.

Daily intake of fresh life energy and chlorophyll directly from nature is very important. You should try to consume at least some of it every day. Optimally, it makes up a large part of your diet. No matter where you live, you'll find something. If you're on raw food only, not eating wild plants, you might feel week and hungry once in a while.

Go to a health food store or look for an organic farm where you can find fresh fruits, vegetables, lettuce, seeds and nuts. Just try out all the different varieties and see what you prefer.

Of course, you'll consume everything without salt, pepper, vinegar and oil. Use lemon, avocado and fresh herbs such as parsley, dill, cilantro or chives in order to enhance the flavour.

It is a delight, I promise.

Have you ever seen a monkey putting oil, salt and pepper on its leaves? It's a very unnatural thing. All kinds of oil are made by humans. Oil as we use it, doesn't occur in nature in pure form. If you use it in salads, it deposits a film on the lettuce's leaves and associated digestive programs get troubled.

From now on, abstain from salt entirely. It is a matter of pure habit.

If you'd drink a certain amount of dissolved salt in water, you die. Try to bear that in mind. How can something be good for you that you could actually die from?

In this form, nature doesn't provide it for you. Species appropriate nutrition excellently gives you everything you need.

Believe me – you don't need salt if you nourish yourself in a species appropriate way.

Uncooked food is full of mineral salts, be it magnesium, sodium, calcium or potassium; precisely like our system requires. Consuming common salt is a threat to your health, especially sodium chloride, meaning sodium and toxic chlorine.

Salt increases the amount of water within your body. Salt calls for fluids and therefore creates excess water in you. It can even damage renal functions.

I get so incredibly thirsty once I eat something salty. It is really incredible how straining it is, but we are all addicted to it. Salt is a flavour carrier.

Salt is so hostile, it even stops natural processes of decay. This was the only reason why it got into our diet to begin with. It was introduced in order to preserve meat, to make it transportable. What have we done with it hundreds of years later?

If your health has true worth to you, remove salt from your food, as it was originally intended. As a natural consequence, you will sweat less and have a more pleasant smell. You will also stop feeling constantly thirsty.

Remember, being a flavouring agent, salt can be found in almost every edible product. How convenient we don't eat any processed stuff anymore, but only natural food. We therefore don't have to deal with this problem any longer.

We are now moving on to another product that should be totally avoided. The matter is about refined sugar. Sugar, whether it is white, brown or in a syrup form, highly weakens your immune system. It rots your teeth and promotes many serious diseases such as diabetes or gastro-intestinal ailments. Sugar impairs your brain. It affects clear mental thinking. As already mentioned, your immune system is mostly affected by the intake of sugar.

It is completely irrelevant what kind of sugar you're using. If it is processed, it damages. Only in the natural compound of a fruit, can you enjoy the food's sweetness without restraint. You can even nibble on sugar cane, which is very tasty. All these incredible fruits are given to you by nature, so that you can eat your fill.

It is important to bear in mind that sugar is contained in almost every product, showing up under different names. This is also the case with products not even tasting sweet. Look closely.

From now on, completely eliminate sugar of your life, including products containing it.

At the beginning you might feel an irresistible craving. If you feel the need to eat something sweet, reach for some unsulphurized, organic dried fruit such as raisins, dates or figs. Fall back on them only in exceptional cases. Always eat little dried fruit, if at all. Your greediness for sweets will totally decrease after a short time period, promised! All the fruit you are going to eat will be sweet enough. Trust me chocolate addicts, the languor will disappear by itself with the passage of time. Then, someday you'll look back and all you can do is shake your head, thinking how you could ever eat all that.

Honey isn't intended for human beings either. It therefore shouldn't be eaten. It is meant for bees and not for you. Honey serves the bee colony as a food and as a store of energy in order to survive long periods without having any food intake from outside. Human honey production has weakened the natural defences of the bee's population, bringing serious consequences. If there aren't any more bees left, which already happened in some parts of the world, it is likely that our lives will also come to an end. We depend on their pollination work in order to get food. Animals and their products depend on it. They, too, have to eat something.

Think about it.

Besides, how would you actually get closer to a wild bees' nest in nature without protective clothing to wear and not sustaining great harm?

Use clear thinking.

Realize what is intended for you by nature and what is not.

From now on, you don't even need to go to a common supermarket. How pleasant! It saves you time and hassle. No matter what you're going to buy, take a very close look at the product first. Realizing it contains more than one ingredient, you can put it back on the shelf.

If you're still going to enter a common supermarket, then move yourself to its organic section straight away in order to buy fruit, salad, vegetables, seeds and nuts. Try to get all other food from daily walks in nature (i.e. from the forest and meadow). It's also best to eat everything right on the spot, directly from the source.

Of course, you need to be a bit careful while foraging. You can eat a lot from nature, but not everything.

Each climate zone has its edible plants. Get yourself some books on wild plants and start to study their edible qualities. It's fun to become more familiar with your environment. You'll be amazed to see so many edible plants do exist. Another easy way is taking a one day class on edible wild plants in your area, for example at a community college, forester or nature club.

At first, keep the few poisonous plants in mind. You're now on the safe side of life.

You'll see that soon you'll be a small master on this subject and many people, your family and friends

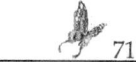

included, will want to be led around in forest and meadow. It will give a lot of pleasure to everyone. A variety of delicious wild plants do exist, tasting good right off the bat.

Eat simple and natural, as often and as much as you want.

You'll never be too fat or too thin.

Don't forget to exercise in a species appropriate way.

Don't worry; I am going to explain this subject a little bit later.

If you're just starting to change your diet, it can be helpful to always carry a small amount of healthy food with you in case you went out and start to feel hungry. Initially put some nuts or fruit into your bag or car so you won't grab onto other things when feeling the urgent need to eat. Later on, species appropriate nutrition will be a natural way of life for you.

Try to eat many leaves and lots of tropical fruits in general. It is helpful to consume food containing plenty of fat, like avocado, nuts and seeds. You'll be amazed how nourished and satisfied you'll feel.

Don't let yourself be put off.

Don't get scared if people start to show their concern, trying to talk you out of this. Full of worries, they'll ask you to stop and be reasonable again. They have never tried this way of life, so how can they judge? They follow a certain lifestyle because others have told them to do so.

Do you also believe anything people have told you, anything that got inoculated into your mind and now you are following it blindly?

Start to think on your own. Find out what things are really about.

Why don't you give a new lifestyle a try, just half a year or less? You can still swing back again if it doesn't seem right, don't you think so?

You might have to process all of this a little bit.

To give you a small break, I am now going to describe how it felt to me when I changed my diet:

*Being confronted with such new information, I mostly just sat there and looked dumbfounded.*

*Somehow everything sounded so clear and logical. Still, I had a critical view and remained in disbelief. Wasn't this all a bit exaggerated?*

*I couldn't deny my life was marked with suffering and disease. I also had tried almost everything in order to get better. Finally, I thought to myself, "What the heck. I am just going to try. I've got nothing to lose. I'll try the whole thing just for one week and observe what happens.*

I should be able to keep some discipline, at least for one week."

I made a clear decision and started to give this new lifestyle a try, just for one week.

It was so difficult to switch my eating habits, especially in the first week! Wasn't food the only thing remaining of the little pleasures and joy in my miserable life?

I gathered all motivation I had left and began to change my diet day by day.

It was wintertime and I was supposed to go outside with my immune system?

I gave it a shot.

I resolved to stop consuming salt and sugar right away. I decided to eat only very little cooked food or other processed items. As far as possible, I wanted to feed myself fresh and unadulterated food.

At the beginning, this was a very difficult thing to do. It felt like being in some sort of withdrawal. I was so dependent on sensations of taste and I missed feeling heavily satiated. These days I would call these feelings 'gluttony' if I thought about it. I was addicted to flavour, rather than just simply nourishing myself.

One night I even dreamt of flying noodles. In my dreams I could grasp them. I fantasized of cakes and potato chips as well as hearty meals. I missed bread, rice and salt, feeling constantly hungry. I was stunned, "One week, that's not a lot! What was that? That could certainly not be it. Come on. You are going to endure this!"

You wouldn't believe how much I wanted to eat a 'real meal' and maybe a dessert afterwards, just a little piece of chocolate, if only a very tiny one. I was greedy to satisfy my palate's desires.

In order to satisfy my craving for a 'dessert', my girlfriend handed me a dried fig instead. That was helpful.

Apparently, it was all a matter of habits.


Despite all pain of renunciation, within days I was already noticing that something was happening to me. Something started to change.

In the beginning I was feeling chilly when taking my 'meals', but no, that wasn't really true. I felt fresh! This kind of inner feeling had been unknown to me so far and I was rating it as feeling cold.

I felt this freshness, a life force flowing into all limbs. This had given me goose bumps in the beginning.

After three days, a friend of mine made some random comments about my appearance, finally asking me why I had such rosy cheeks. I appeared somehow differently. I looked into the mirror. Yes, it was true. I was looking a little bit different than I used to.

It wasn't just my skin's appearance that had changed; my eyes also got a different expression. I looked more alive.

*I started to reduce my medication dose. To my surprise, that didn't worsen my symptoms. I was amazed to see that. Usually I felt worse when I tried to reduce my medication intake. The pain would get so unbearable that I really needed the drugs.*

*Now, however, it was different. I gradually let go of the medication I took and while doing this, I even started to feel better. I really thought a miracle was happening. It was unbelievable.*

*In the morning, I ate lots of fruit and by saying this, I really mean a lot, not just two apples. Later on I put some bananas into my bag and walked to the nearest park.*

*There I was, armed with my bananas; ready to eat straight from nature. I looked around. Being wintertime, there were little plants to choose from, but even the plants I got to see I knew nothing about. I couldn't even name them. What kind of tree was that? What is the name for the bush over there? Here, these tiny green plants on the ground, what are they all about?*

*I was shocked.*

*I could feel how far I had drifted away from nature. I had got to the point that I couldn't even name trees, shrubs and little plants that I was surrounded with for more than 30 years.*

*It amazed me and gave me motivation to learn more about my environment.*

*In the end, I also wanted to have some kind of selection on my new menu.*

*Did I really know nothing at all?*

*I saw a few brambles, nettles, mosses and ferns. That's what I had to make do with at first.*

*I began to pick a little bit from each plant and just put them into my mouth. Small nettle leaves I wrapped into larger bramble's leaves, so that they wouldn't sting and burn my tongue.*

*At first I had to overcome some kind of resistance in order to eat wild plants, but it also amused me to do something that appeared so completely different to me. Initially the plants tasted unusually bitter.*

*Human beings have taken most bitter flavours from their diet, thinking life is more pleasant without it, even though it is unnatural. Bitter substances, however, are important and certainly belong into our system. Nature is just full of them and I don't see any animal complaining.*

*Since then, bitter substances have become pleasant to me. It's all a question of habit.*

*To make it easier, my teacher Franz Konz used to show us a good way to eat bitter leaves. Together with the leaf I put a piece of fruit into my mouth so that the unusual taste and sensation got more pleasant. I chewed it all together, realizing it wasn't that bad at all. It tasted pretty good, a little unusual, but not too bad.*

I continued to walk around and tried out a few more plants. I smiled at fellow people walking their dogs, giving me an occasionally strange or surprising look. I just said 'hi' to them. I had to become a little bit looser. Often-times I ended up having some real interesting conversations. To my surprise, while foraging I met plenty of people showing a lot of openness and interest in what I was doing. Some of them even told me where to find the best berries and fruit trees in the area.

Before I went home, I made sure to take some plants with me. I planned on eating them later that day or by the next morning.

One evening, after searching for food in the forest, I lay down at home in order to rest. All of a sudden tears started to flow all over my face. I was crying.

It wasn't sadness that was causing this flow of tears. Deep feelings of relief, feelings of redemption and gratitude came upon me. I felt connected to everything.

What an overwhelming feeling.

I felt like creation suddenly swung wide open, catching and embracing me with open arms.

From that moment I knew something of what I was doing was right. I therefore wanted to give it a real shot. I decided to try out this new way of life for three months. I made a conscious commitment.

*In spite of old habits and major concerns of many fellow people, I wanted to continue doing the things that had just begun.*

*"Now you have become mad", they said. Doctors and friends wanted to lock me away for my own safety.*

*In the second week, I decided to leave behind the little bit of cooked food I was still eating. I also stopped consuming bread that I was still eating on occasion. Sunflower seeds went very well with salad and I imagined them being a good substitute for bread.*

*What was there to lose anyway? I really wanted to try out this method exactly. I, therefore, made no exceptions.*

*I remained steadfast, seeing everyone around me eating, walking by tempting smells of bakeries and snack bars. I'd be lying, saying it was easy. It was very difficult, but it was worth the hold out. I trusted that my habits would change. I also got motivated by feeling the clarity of already having gained so much progress on my health in such a short time. I felt better every day. This feeling was worth any discipline.*

*I trusted that man is a creature of habit and that everything takes its time. I decided just to go ahead and so I did.*

*Very soon I was finally able to sleep again, after many years of the worst sleeping disorder.*

*I knew this was also a result of the plants I was consuming. Like the plants, my system started to calm down at night. I ate them, they were inside of me and thus I came to rest. I picked up their rhythm, which is entirely focused on the sun's availability.*

*Over time I realized how much I had clung to food. I noticed many of my fellow human beings did so too. Food is a big part of our social system. I could see almost everyone strongly defending their favourite food.*

*Why couldn't we just eat something else instead?*

*Would the food's flavour really matter if we needed to survive?*

*If we are hungry, then why not eat to simply nourish ourselves?*

*I had been unconsciously eating to satisfy some kind of hunger, but not that of my stomach. I realized often-times I was eating out of boredom, stress, loneliness, and pure habit, in order to find comfort or simply just to distract myself. Since I couldn't do this any longer, I immediately began to feel when something was wrong in my life. It was now necessary to look at things. It was on me to find real solutions, rather than just grabbing food. I started to recognize my own truth and got more aware of my real longings and grievances. Things began to change. My life began to improve and to clarify.*

In the following, I would like to explain a few more things about species appropriate nutrition, which is well-worth knowing in my opinion.

All organisms on this planet are designed for a specific habitat and a particular climate.

Would this also be the case for us?

Would human beings, as creatures of nature, really be able to survive in ice and snow, without civilization?

Could they live in colder seasons, without housing, heating and warm clothes?

If so, what would they eat?

Even in areas where there's little water and hardly any vegetation, it is questionable whether human beings would survive relying on original conditions given by creation.

Humanity's origin was found to be in Africa. There, our story began. The great apes are our relatives and live in harmony with nature. They can still be found exclusively in those areas with warm climates and areas rich in vegetation, arranged for them by creation.

Only by turning away from their original programming, by separating from nature, man was able to penetrate into other climatic areas. Cultural inventions like tools, made humans settle down all over the planet, and everything else took its course. These days we can find cities hosting millions of people.

It is as it is. The human population increased to an unnaturally high degree. We spread all over the world. Our planet is suffering and also a vast majority of us humans don't feel that well. Diseases come upon the world's civilisation. No one seems to be spared.

What can we do, here and now to still meet our system's needs no matter the circumstances? On the diet level, it is of the utmost importance to take fresh, raw food directly from nature. It's good to repeat this as often as possible.

It is also useful to consider our origin. In addition to daily 'direct intake', it's good to consume food from the tropics.

Due to stronger sun exposure, tropical fruits often-times are more nutritious and saturating than the fruit of colder climates.

A climatic approach also leads us to consider mealtimes. If we take a look at our related apes, we can observe that they finish their food intake by late afternoon.

They then prepare an individual sleeping place and slowly come to rest.

They follow this special rhythm because every day at 6pm it becomes dark in the tropics and that can happen very quickly.

Because of their physical features, primates are made to rest when it's dark. How could we see when there's no light around us? We can't see at night. How should we walk around, looking for food or doing other things, if we can't even see our hands in front of us?

Nature is very simple. It is showing you how to behave properly. It takes your hand, if you allow it to do so. Your digestive system isn't made to consume food at night.

Everything is connected. In the principles of creation, the same perfection is always visible.

If, for us, eating after 6pm is actually not possible, we shouldn't act against nature's laws and do it anyway.

Quality of sleep and nightly recovery can interfere with eating late, especially if you're a very sensitive person.

From eating late, your body has to digest during the night instead of during the day. That is not part of its original program. Thus, you might not get a good rest.

Just stop eating when it is about to become dark outside. Don't consume any food at least after 7pm. You don't feel full and satiated? So what! Try it out. Don't judge these feelings as something bad. Just do it.

Sensations of feeling hungry or satiated will change.

In the beginning, you'll probably miss the usual 'heavy' feeling of satiety you're used to. You start to think: "Somehow something is missing," although you have eaten a lot of fresh food and nothing more could fit in your belly.

I'd like to briefly tell another story of mine:

*I liked traveling to Central America and prior to changing my diet, I always loved to eat typical dishes, consisting of rice, beans, fish and salad. It always agreed with me and I felt strong and satiated.*

*Years later, I travelled again over there. I got very tempted and ordered a meal, despite of my new lifestyle. It still tasted good to me.*

*Suddenly, I felt something very unpleasant in my stomach. Instead of having just eaten a meal, I felt I had swallowed two large stones, now lying inside of me: one on the left, and one on the right side of my belly. All of the sudden I started to feel heavily tired and with a lot of effort I managed to drag myself straight into my hotel.*

*I lay down at once and within a few seconds I fell asleep for a couple of hours.*

Let's take a brief look at what to drink.

If you eat processed food, of course you have to drink plenty of fluids.

In most cases, common food is salted and contains little liquid. When I consume processed food, I feel very thirsty too, and then, of course, I also drink more.

If you're eating fresh food only, you'll feel less thirsty and automatically drink less. That's all right. Fresh food consists largely of bound water. Whether it is a cucumber, lettuce, dandelion or rose petals, all of these foods have a water content of over 95 percent. Even fresh apples consist of 85 percent water, bananas about 75 percent. Is it a coincidence that our muscle tissue is also made of 75 percent water?

Our fluid requirement depends on the food we eat and can therefore never be defined on a general level. Species appropriate nutrition already contains most of the liquid your body requires. Eating naturally, you automatically have a high intake of liquid. It happens precisely, exactly as it is made for you. This can never be imitated by any human.

Trust your body.

If you feel thirsty, drink still water at room temperature only. Only once in a while take juices and only those squeezed on your own. Drink them only if you absolutely need to. Store bought juices usually originate in factories. Whatever promising information you read on the package, just ask yourself, "How can those juices be fresh"? Consider also all the pesticides and additives you'll probably consume with them.

It is also unnatural to drink something heated. Which creature on this planet does something like that? Just think of all those tea beverages recommended to drink while being sick. Somehow I never got better more quickly and I used to be sick all the time, especially during wintertime.

Why do we drink tea? Do we believe there are some magical herbs in it? The herbs are already dead anyway, does pouring hot water over them cause some magical essence to be released? In addition, hot substances enter your gastrointestinal tract and thus more micro-organisms get destroyed. Remember, being in symbiosis with them is very important for your health.

Of all the drinks, alcohol and coffee might be the ones that can damage you most. You being dependent on them, should give you a warning right away. They are unnatural human products, not doing you any good in the long run.

Among caffeine, coffee has an acid effect. It's that simple.

It irritates your stomach and intestines, making it vulnerable to all kinds of diseases.

It stops your system from digesting food in a proper way, ending up with serious health problems.

Do you suffer from bloating, abdominal cramps, gastritis, gas, acid reflux or heartburn?

Does irritable bowel syndrome, constipation or diarrhoea sound familiar?

Could coffee play also a role in colon cancer?

Wake up for real!

Coffee's laxative effects overstimulate your digestive system, making the stomach's contents pass too quickly. Going to the bathroom often times is related to a cup of coffee. Unfortunately, this quick passing has other consequences too. Less nutrients get absorbed from not being able to properly break down food. Highly important life substances like iron, calcium, zinc, magnesium or vitamin b will be lacking.

In addition, the roasting process of coffee beans produces Acetylamide, well known as a cancer causing substance.

Drinking coffee increases muscle tension, blood pressure and heart rate by releasing stress hormones like cortisol and adrenalin. It makes your system feel like being in a real emergency situation. You get highly alert, gathering all resources of energy in order to face the 'danger'. You put yourself in a state of fight or flight.

Where is the tiger though?

Do you really need to fight for your survival all the time, facing tigers all day long?

Wouldn't we rather have to do that only once in a while?

You're constantly on, constantly poisoning yourself.

Physically, coffee puts you under constant stress, even though you don't notice and you seem to work well. Of course you don't realize. It's obvious your life is not in danger at all. Getting 'down' you start to feel tired, exhausted, being easily irritated and there you go for the next cup of coffee.

What a threat to your health!

How can you treat yourself so badly?

Don't you love yourself at all?

Drinking coffee is not natural at all.

Even though it seems like a waste of time to me, let us also briefly discuss drinking alcohol in any form.

Drinking alcohol weakens your immune system to a tremendous amount, especially if it comes to viral infections and tumour cells. Being in the body, the alcohol is broken down to acetaldehyde, a highly toxic substance, causing damage to your DNA. There's no cancer unless DNA is altered.

The risk of cancer through alcohol consumption is well proven. Breast cancer, bowel cancer and oral cancers are just a few.

Alcohol damages your brain by harming neural connections. It is highly involved when it comes to loosing memory skills. It causes gastritis and ulcers in your stomach. It can also lead to high blood pressure, heart failure or stroke. Will you really enjoy your next drink not caring about yourself at all?

In men consumption of alcohol lowers sperm's quality and quantity. More estrogen and less testosterone can be found in the body. In women, abilities to conceive are affected.

Alcohol simply makes you fat. Even though it is high on calories, it makes you eat more because sugar gets stored away.

Isn't that all kind of disgusting?

Alcohol is toxic. It makes you lose fluids, causing headaches and loss of minerals.

It damages your liver. It's totally inappropriate.

As you can see, both alcohol and coffee can harm you to a high degree.

Stop drinking them.

Many of us cling to coffee in order to be awake. We got used to drinking our beer or wine to relax or just to socialize.

Just give it a try and stop this habit. As a result you might realize how you're feeling for real.

What a way of life we got used to.

Wouldn't you rather be healthy?

Don't you want to decide for yourself what you really want to consume? Let go of blindly reacting to habits and desires, without regard for the consequences. If you're tired, then ask yourself why.

Instead of grabbing some coffee, just try something different to wake you up. You could just jump up and down, run a lap or do a headstand, which, believe me, you can learn.

Just choose to give it a shot and do things differently.

Do it for yourself, for your health. There's something waiting for you that might feel even better than things you're currently experiencing.

From now on, only drink still water at room temperature if you feel thirsty at all. Inquire about the water's ingredients you are consuming and avoid those with lots of chlorine. Don't drink too much water out of plastic bottles either.

Ideally consume spring water.

It's a sad irony that even though we live on a planet extremely rich in water, we still have to worry about where to find any that is safe to drink.

Let's talk about food again.

It is important to eat in tranquillity and peace.

Take your time.

Don't do anything else while eating.

Avoid big conversations, don't read your newspaper; have the radio and TV switched off. Your food wants to be absorbed and digested in peace. This already starts by thorough mastication. All essential digestive programs get set in motion right at the beginning.

Avoid eating when being emotional and upset. Never eat in a hurry.

How did life go on with me and species appropriate eating?

Here's how my story continued:

*Three months of 'probation' had passed. Every day I was doing my regular 'health program'. Now and then, I still found it a bit difficult seeing other people eating, but friends and family helped me to remain steadfast.*

*After all these years of suffering, they could witness the positive changes I was experiencing.*

*No, living like that wasn't bad at all. I felt so much better. I actually had become very happy.*

*I really didn't want to break up with these newly acquired habits. They were only three months old, unlike my old habit of 30 plus years. I wanted to cultivate and maintain what had just begun.*

*I was pleased with this new lifestyle. I felt how much good it did to me. I therefore decided to keep going. I really wanted to try it. I wanted to observe its results for a whole year. "It's just one year", I thought.*

*I had lost some weight and it concerned me slightly. However, I trusted everything takes its time and that I'd put on weight again.*

*So it happened. After six months, I automatically started to gain weight again. These days I have my old weight back. It really worked.*

*I never wanted to eat salt, sugar or bread again. I didn't feel like it. I shuddered just thinking of all these finished products. I didn't want to put something like that into my body any longer. Bread reminded me more and more of cardboard or paper packaging. I couldn't see anything nourishing in it, except that it filled the belly. Cooked food served on a plate looked to me as pre-digested mush:*

*limp and flabby.*

*Eating other than fresh food, I immediately felt the consequences. After consuming dairy products, I instantly started to get sinus mucus, which luckily disappeared quickly, just by going back on a natural diet. How pleasant not to feel helpless any longer regarding this coming and going of diseases.*

*After four months, though, I'd had enough. I really wanted to please my spoiled taste buds once in a while, just a little bit. In social affairs my lifestyle was also a bit disturbing sometimes. Nevertheless, I wanted to stick with it. I couldn't imagine doing anything else. It was just too good for me and I felt so clear.*

*I opted for a compromise. Once a week I wanted to make an exception and bring my chattering mind to rest. On occasions, such as invitations, birthdays or just because I wanted to, I ate something different. It was a pleasant experience to taste other kinds of foods, just once in a while. I still avoided consuming any sugar, bread and heavily processed foods. I didn't feel like putting garbage into my body any longer. If I made an exception, then I always chose something light – meals, society considers 'very healthy'.*

*I realized I didn't want to be dogged or hard. With joy I wanted to establish a species appropriate diet into my life. I wanted to create it as an everyday habit for the long run.*

*I stayed awake not to dissolve my habits, but to make sure the exceptions I made remained exceptions.*

*So it was. As already mentioned, I was feeling way too good. It would have been unthinkable to swap this for old patterns.*

*I kept track and stuck with it.*

*If there happened to be many opportunities for making an 'exception', I stuck to fruit and nuts instead, which I would bring with me. Interestingly, most people weren't aversed to that. I was very often asked different kinds of questions, realizing many fellow people found this diet to be quite appealing and worthy of emulation.*

*I missed my old eating habits less every day. It wasn't an option to me any longer. When a year had passed, I took stock. What had happened? What had changed?*

*I didn't take any kind of medication. I was able to move my body and challenge it much more. I finally found some sleep. I was positive and optimistic. I had separated from many things that were not doing me any good.*

*It was clear to me that after reviewing such a positive balance, I decided to stay with this new way of life as long as it would fit and serve me.*

*So far, I haven't encountered any better diet.*

Many times people ask, "What do you actually eat all day and how do you feel full with it?" Below, I'll give you a concrete example of my everyday life, representing a general eating pattern:

First and foremost my diet depends on where I live because it needs to be fresh.

Early in the morning I typically eat fruits and wild plants, plucking them freshly if possible or grabbing some leftovers from the previous day.

Later on I eat some nuts or seeds.

After noon, I mostly eat salad. I take a conventional organic salad, mixing in wild plants, flower petals, cucumber, tomato and lots of fresh herbs like chives, parsley or coriander. Furthermore, I put some lemon over it, sometimes just a few drops of water. I like to eat avocado, carrots or sunflower seeds with salad.

In the evening, I mostly eat fruit and plants.

After 7pm, I stop consuming food, no matter how 'hungry' I feel.

I think we eat too much anyway.

This diet is not associated with a lot of effort because you no longer have to cook or clean a lot of pots and pans afterwards. It's convenient and time saving. No matter where I go, I can always bring something with me. Depending on where I am, I could also forage food right on the spot. I see a certain tree or some edible plant and just go for it. With just a small grasp in the abundance surrounding us, it is possible to absorb fresh life energy, to refresh and nourish our system.

Life is beautiful.

Go and ingest it.

Knowing I will be out the whole day, I prepare myself a meal bag. It could happen that I have to stay inside all day long, at work or in the car. I just take a container of salad with me and also nuts and fruit. I am ready to go. It's that easy.

Finishing this chapter, I'd like to mention another interesting consequence of this type of diet: You're hardly producing any waste.

Almost your entire food garbage can end up on a compost heap and that feels good. Rather than putting more burdens on this planet, from now on your waste is even producing fertile soil.

Isn't that a miracle?

With this kind of lifestyle, you're hurting our planet way less and everything can remain in more peace and harmony. Wasn't that the original plan anyway?

The chapter on a species appropriate diet had to be very detailed because it is the furthest away from common thoughts and daily habits. Approaching this type of diet therefore needed to be illuminated in a very particular and extensive way. The following chapter will talk about species appropriate exercising.

Moving your body in a species appropriate way has the same value for your health and well-being as species appropriate eating. It is even a bit more important. Thus, make sure to read this chapter very closely too.

If you feel this is right, then put it into practice by making it a part of your daily life.

# II. Species appropriate exercise

One thing is certain: Human beings have to move their bodies properly; otherwise there will be problems in the long run. There's just nothing to change that, even though we like our comfort zone and exercise may be inconvenient to us.

Our original programming exists. We have a body that is made to move extensively. If we lived a natural lifestyle, our body would be flexible and agile, full of strength and endurance. All these abilities were given to us in order to live and survive.

When talking about a species appropriate diet, quite a few bits of information have already been given. We are clearer about the nature that we are a part of. As a natural conclusion the following question arises: What kind of movements do we need in order to procure natural food?

Considering we are living beings of nature, we are likely to perform the movements I am going to describe now. We will also talk about exercising in general. At first, it is important basing physical training on the following natural body movements:

Living in nature consists of lots of walking and some running too. We would squat, stretch far up and also reach out to all sides; we would pull ourselves up, push things away or lift them up. We might climb, shim, jump off elevations, balance, crawl and climb over obstacles.

We should do these kinds of movements every day. If we don't, we are following a lifestyle not meeting our natural needs at all. As a result we might feel uncomfortable and sick.

Of course, natural exercising involves much more.

It is very complex. You'll find out yourself when picking plants or berries.

Don't worry, you don't have to go out there into the jungle and jump around like a savage now. Although, I can thoroughly recommend leaving old routines behind like walking on groomed trails. Finally step onto real soil of forest and meadow.

It feels fantastic, so soft and gentle.

It's a real treat, set for us by creation in order to walk and run. How nice not to walk on concrete any longer.

It's not just natural eating leading us to an understanding of species appropriate exercising. Every organism is perfectly equipped in order to perform those kinds of movements, necessary for its specific needs and habitat.

Humans in nature run very fast, or quickly climb up a tree in order to get to safety.

It would be necessary to prepare a place to sleep by using natural resources we'd gather from nature.

We would have babies with us, carrying them close to our bodies. There are no strollers in the wild and even these days you won't see animals putting their young ones into strollers. The little ones are always near an adult's body and well protected by the whole group. The young ones get challenged too. Soon after being born, they learn to maintain a firm grip on a family member's body, otherwise they would fall down.

In everything you are doing, ask yourself, "Is it natural?"

If you have any doubts about your lifestyle, or if you're not feeling well, you can always ask yourself this question, finding help within its answer.

Which of your daily physical movements are still natural?


In modern society our body mostly acts in a very unnatural way. We mainly exercise too little or do sports that are one-sided.

You should walk, run, jump, stretch and reach out, crawl, lie, climb, pull, push and much more.

Walking sufficiently and getting a good long stretch are things particularly missing in everyday life. This, however, should be your main activity and not sitting in chairs, couches, driving cars or other unilateral strains like standing straight or holding a jackhammer all day long.

If you're constantly having injuries, something's wrong with the sport you're doing. Think about long-term damages too. Your musculoskeletal system suffers from those kinds of sports. Ask yourself, "Would I really perform these physical movements living naturally?"

Walk more, but do it on natural ground and not on concrete. While walking in the forest, you might see a branch above you. Why don't you jump up and just let your body hang on it? Pull yourself up to the branch, so your muscles get stronger.

From now on move your body in a natural and harmonious way.

Most sports are not adapted to our physical system. They disturb its harmonious processes and in the long run, its functionality. Certain sports stress our bodies because they're not appropriate for our species. They are virtually not useful for our survival. Whether it is playing tennis, soccer, basketball, doing judo, skiing, rowing, running a marathon or performing other one-sided sports, it can become a strain to your body. Our system is not created for that kind of stress and you might feel this sooner or later through pain, injuries, inflammation or wear. Your body sends out signals. It shows you that it doesn't do it any good. It asks you to desist, so that it can continue to function without interference.

Moving your body in a species appropriate way, you'll have no problems. Life is beautiful and comfortable. You feel good. You feel better every day. You're experiencing becoming more fit and agile.


Nevertheless, it's good to have some fun too.

Try to find a good balance in the way you exercise.

Generally said, it is highly important to move your body sufficiently and regularly.

Ideally perform natural exercises on a daily base except you should take one day 'off', meaning you don't do any physical training during this particular day.

Regeneration and relaxation play the same important part in effective training like active training itself.

The most important thing, however, is to stick with your training. Stay in motion your whole life, until you've reached the final end.

As previously mentioned, it is important to walk and run.

Take a look. How is your walking style? Do you walk upright and still relaxed? Does your foot unroll from heel to ball of foot? What kind of shoes are you wearing?

Now and then try to run, at least sometimes.

Pay attention to your running style. If you want to understand what a healthy running style really implies, then ask yourself the following question: What if we didn't wear shoes?

While running, take small steps.

Make sure to touch the ground bales first, instead of landing on your heels like most amateur runners do.

This unnatural running behaviour is caused by modern footwear, distorting natural movements of barefoot running.

Get thin, flexible running shoes or so-called five-finger shoes, being the closest to barefoot running.

If possible, go barefoot sometimes. That's your natural behaviour.

Natural running is very well described by Christopher McDougall in *Born to run*.

Don't give up and don't be too hard on yourself.

Do a step by step approach. Be patient, but keep going. Do something.

From now on feel comfortable while performing natural exercises, even if they seem exhausting to you.

Are you putting tension into muscles you actually don't need for this specific exercise?

Do you have unnecessary tension in your face or hands while working out?

What is your breath doing?

Do you continue to breathe or are you actually holding your breath?

Your system needs oxygen, especially while exercising. Breathe!

Make an attempt and deliberately decide to sit less. Your favourite sofa secretly might cause you a lot of discomfort.

Move all seating items out of your sight for a while. Observe how much time you actually spend sitting during the day. Even driving a car is a seated affair. The percentage of time we spend sitting is more than enough.

Sometimes it might be inevitable to sit, like at work. If this is the case, then don't continue to also sit during your break, and in particular not in your spare time. No wonder so many people suffer from back pain. Lie, squat, stand or walk instead. If you happen to sit, seat yourself at the chair's front edge.

Hold your upper body straight and firmly anchor both legs in an angle of 90 degrees on the ground.

Attitude and sitting habits will change. You just have to do it for a while. Never forget about performing species appropriate exercise either. There's always time. It's a priority thing.

Specific muscle training can be helpful, especially in the beginning. It also makes you gain weight. If necessary go to a gym every once in a while. If you're just starting to change your lifestyle, it might be useful. Your whole body is about to change and all your muscles want to grow. You'll be much stronger. In nature, muscles get used every single day.

Considering everything in its entirety, we can realize creation is a miracle. Look at how we were created and how one thing interlocks with another. Some of our main lymph nodes are located at the groin and near the armpits. Nothing is random. They are located in spots, where our body naturally moves a lot, rather than on the tibia or on the head. Some of the main lymph nodes are located exactly where they naturally stay in motion, so that they can work well and detoxify our system. To walk, run or squat our legs, to bend and stretch our arms, does just that. Everything is perfectly arranged.

It is automatically regulated if we stick to our place in creation.

While exercising, you'll start to breathe deeper, so that your body can be supplied with oxygen. When doing your workout outside in nature, healthy air automatically enters the lungs and cardiovascular system. From there, all your cells get refreshed with oxygen of the highest quality.

Move your body extensively for at least two hours a day. If you're feeling a bit insecure and you don't know how to move properly, it might be helpful to get some information at first. A very good resource to learn some healthy stretching and strengthening exercises would be certain movements from Pilates, Yoga or therapeutic trainings. As already mentioned, you don't need to climb trees all day long, constantly swinging from branch to branch.

Additionaly, you can take classes held by professional trainers too.

You can also do your workout at home, taking fitness DVDs or videos you can find online for help and motivation. This can be seen as occasional exceptions from exercising outdoors.

Whatever you decide to do: keep in mind that you should treat your body in a holistic way. It's important to stretch and strengthen your muscles, but that's not all. Your heart and your state of endurance should also be strengthened.

I therefore repeat: Walk and run a lot, otherwise you'll treat yourself too one-sided.

Franz Konz provides wonderfully illustrated exercises for species appropriate training, and they're quite inspiring.

When exercising, always consider and appreciate your whole body. Take care of yourself by moving all body parts: Head, face, jaw, neck and also shoulders. Train your arms, take care of elbows and wrists; stretch and strengthen all your fingers.

Keep your spine agile and smooth. Train abdominal and back muscles.

Your body wants to be entirely seen.

Take care of the pelvic floor, hips and buttocks. Strengthen and stretch your legs. Pay attention to your small but all important foot muscles. Stretch your toes to all sides and rub your feet.

Your feet carry you all your life and we force them into unnatural shoes. Your whole posture is based on them. Give them some attention.

Massage your scalp a bit.

Loosen up legs and arms by shaking them for a while.

If not exercising, let go.

Try to get back in contact with your body. A very helpful exercise can be guided 'journeys', so called body-scans.

Take a look at children being on a playground. It's an amazing spectacle. It is so impressive to see them dangle on horizontal bars, preferably upside down and then they even swing to and fro!

"What a pity," I thought to myself.

"I am so out of practice and I now no longer dare doing that kind of stuff."

I realized it had nothing to do with my age. Regarding my natural design, I was genetically still capable of performing great movements, but training was missing. Muscles and neural connections were totally lacking, out of pure neglect.

Children intuitively know how to move in a naturally appropriate way.

Join in moving with your children, imitating everything they suggest. This will certainly end up being very funny for all of you.

Intuitive natural body movements and the simple joy of it have, unfortunately, been forced out of us by society very early. By the age of six or even sooner, we start to visit this institution called school, being forced to sit perfectly still against our natural program.

What kind of human education is that or should I better use the word 'domestication', which the author, Don Miguel Ruiz, prefers to call the process of socialization?

If a child is not able to sit still, this will be handled as a 'problem'. Humans' brains and bodies are made to move and not to sit. With this type of education, we're literally forcing both down onto the chair. Transition already starts at an early age.

In the following I'll talk about my own experiences. This time I'm going to describe how it felt to me approaching species appropriate exercising.

*Coinciding with changing my diet, I also tried to challenge my body a little bit more, even though I had strong doubts about it.*

*I always had bad experiences attempting to challenge my body and so I was critical trying to exercise again. What could I do with all these aching muscles and joints? Trying to exercise always felt like a burden on my aching body and doing it always produced more pain and inflammation.*

*When I started, I could only walk about 200 yards.*

*I wanted to make it at least to the next city park.*

*I wore knee braces and walked in a limping manner.*

*Once I reached the park, I stepped on a grassy area and did some light stretching and strengthening exercises.*

*I decided to go there daily for the next few days.*

*I moved my body as best as possible in a species appropriate way for about two hours a day. To my surprise it didn't create more pain. This was absolutely contrary to my expectations. I was amazed seeing my body move like this. In a very slow and gradual manner, I tried to increase the workout's intensity.*

*Sometimes I had to experience little setbacks, but they never lasted long. It really took off with my well-being.*

*I also learned how to approach these setbacks properly. I realized, metaphorically, that even though I was going three steps forward and one step backwards, I was still going two steps forward. This adds up to a tremendous amount of forward progress in time.*

*After a short time, I managed to walk longer distances. I was amazed and happy. I was able to join others for a walk and keep up with them.*

*In the past, people always had to wait for me, I struggled keeping pace.*

*While doing species appropriate exercises, I always made sure not to walk or run on concrete, but instead on natural* ground. Now and then I saw a tree's branch, inviting me to jump up and let my body dangle and stretch. There I was, hanging off a tree, swinging back and forth. I tried to pull myself up to it or lift my legs around the branch I was holding onto.

I gradually explored my urban environmental forest by walking and running cross-country through nature, over meadows, roots and tree trunks.

Sometimes I even got lost in our urban forest.

I found it a bit annoying, but it also amused me. In the end, I was still in civilization, where nature stops at a certain point. Luckily, I always got home somehow. It taught me to be more humble and take precautions for further adventures.

While exploring the urban forest, I looked for opportunities to challenge my body. I climbed over small obstacles and jumped off small elevations right into soft leaves of the forest's ground. It was beautiful. It reminded me of my childhood days and as I looked back, I realized how easy and pain free these movements were back then.

Now, however, I had to find my way back.

I really wanted to move my body like I did in the past.

I had to approach the whole thing slowly and deliberately if I didn't want to hurt myself.

Once again, it amazed me to see how far my body and all its capacities had drifted away from its natural state. My *musculoskeletal system was no longer prepared for these types of movements. I slowly had to get used to them again.*

*Instead of meeting friends in town, I took them with me into the forest. They were very interested in what I was doing and to my surprise they wanted to taste some of my favourite plants.*

*Once, we even climbed up a small tree. There we were, having a nice conservation in the forest while sitting in the branches of a tree. We were not in some kind of bar around the corner.*

*Being an adult, it was funny to do things like that, but wasn't that our ailments' main cause? Of course I got strange looks from others doing stuff like that. On the other hand, many people came up to me and wanted to know what exactly I was doing and why. They liked it; especially after talking to me and realizing I wasn't a maniac at all. I could feel there was a forgotten longing slumbering in many of them. It was about being embedded in nature, but society's pressure of conformity, other people's expectations and the pursuit of a behaviour considered as normal, do create big blockades.*

*What do other people think of me?*

*We always want to be loved and accepted by our fellow human beings.*

*We are afraid of being rejected.*

While I was at home, I also did some stretching and strengthening exercises. I decided to see it as body hygiene like brushing my teeth. It was necessary and simply good for me, even though it required some discipline. I really wanted to specifically train and strengthen my muscles after all these years of not using them. I therefore decided to go to a gym. It was good for a while, but in the end I preferred to exercise outdoors.

Sometimes I needed variety and inspiration during training. As I wasn't looking for hassle and cost, I just got some second hand fitness DVDs or watched free classes online. I made sure to enjoy nature afterwards. Whenever I felt like doing something new or different, I was now able to have choices: today I will do some yoga, tomorrow Pilates and next week I might try a boxing workout. I had a huge selection of fitness DVDs and used ones were so cheap to get.

At the library I borrowed books on strength and endurance training. I used the information I got from these books and applied it to my own knowledge of species appropriate exercising.

I learned a lot and it was helpful many times. I still made sure not to take over other peoples' knowledge without checking first. The given advice had to be natural and appropriate for my species.

I felt better every day.

Once in a while though, I was experiencing a few setbacks. They made me realize to treat myself in a more gentle and loving way. Besides the training, I had to allow my body time for relaxation and regeneration.

I was so happy being able to move my body again that I was tempted to try out other sports, sports I loved doing before I got sick. In moderation it was possible and I really enjoyed it, but with time I felt my pain was increasing again. At first it bothered me, but I wasn't surprised either. I understood that by performing these kinds of sports, I was moving my system in an unnatural way. I wouldn't get well in the long run. My body quickly showed me what it needed and I acknowledged it for my own benefit. I wanted to feel good. I therefore decided to perform other sports only once in a while and mainly do species appropriate exercises.

It was great to understand things.

I no longer felt helpless regarding my suffering.

I also noticed how much time we spend seated in society. I was tired of all this sitting. I felt that it caused me pain. I decided to consciously observe my moving and sitting behaviour in everyday life and to sit as little as possible.

I said to myself, "How much time do we all spend sitting! If I get tired of moving around or if I simply don't want to move at all, then I'm going to find another solution.

*I just stand and lean my body on a wall, crouch, lie down, sometimes on the floor."*

*This wasn't easy at the beginning.*

*Like most people, I had become quite stiff from living an adult life.*

*After eight months, I left my knee bandages behind.*

*I had been using them for running or walking long distances. One day I accidentally lost them while hiking. Since then, I have never used knee bandages again.*

*It felt like a miracle to me, because since age 13, I had always suffered from knee pain. I understood very clearly one thing leads another: Having a species appropriate diet, I was able to train my musculoskeletal system. By challenging my body, step by step I started to build up muscles and strengthen myself.*

Nature is very smart. All living beings are perfectly equipped to survive. Opportunities to rest and to refuel energy are also included. Unfortunately our life drifted away in an uncontrollable way. Yes, we are programmed to save energy and to rest if possible, but we no longer have a natural lifestyle. If we would live in nature, we would be physically very active for the purpose of survival. These days we are designing our lives in a special way. It's mainly about saving physical energy. Our genes, however, haven't changed yet. Our body is not a seat apparatus with a giant head, but a musculoskeletal system with arms and legs. We need to move our body. Every human system is created the same way.

Let's talk about my friend Daniel. Many years ago, he traded an academic career for working in organic gardening. He slept outside in a tent, taking care of fruit trees and vegetables he was surrounded with. Every day he was working outside inhaling fresh air, rain or shine. When he started to work as a gardener, often-times he thought about not being able to perform all this physical work any longer. He initially felt quite exhausted. These days, he feels as good as can be. It's been more than 15 years now. He describes himself as strong and fit. He says he wouldn't feel any pain in his body. He would never be sick, but instead he felt completely well.

After telling me all that, he just looked at me and said, "At this point in my life, I started to understand. Living outside, not owning a car, but walking a lot and having plenty of other physical activity actually corresponds with human nature."

Indeed, I didn't have any doubts seeing both, his strong body and his relaxing peaceful personality.

I also have another friend, Marc.

I saw him every day at noon. Living in the tropics, this was an hour where no one could walk a single step without getting hit by the heat. He was jogging for several miles along the beach, holding stones in his hands. I was wondering why he would do such a thing. One day I talked to him and asked him about it. He told me his story. He said that he had suffered from colon cancer. He had sold everything he had owned and he would now live in a modest cottage in nature. Every morning he would start his day at 5am doing yoga and meditation. Then he would go for a 7 mile run. In the afternoon he would ride his bicycle for about 60 miles up in the mountains. In between he would work and take care of his son.

"With this kind of lifestyle, I cured myself from cancer." At least, that's what he told me.

I told him about my diet, and that I would do some fasting from time to time. He answered, "I don't need all that, because what I'm doing, that's my fasting."

Indeed, his body must be in a constant state of detoxification, cleansing and renewal.

I agreed and every time he was running by I waved at him.

These are very specific examples. You don't necessarily need to live like that. Nevertheless, even if you're barely able to move your body, or if someday you find yourself stuck in such a situation, move whatever you can. It might be just one eye, one finger or a toe. It doesn't matter.

Keep in motion, always.


I liked talking to elderly people who appear fit and healthy.

Once I had a small conversation with an old man. He was tall and slender, grinning like a child. All of the sudden from standing erect, he went down to the floor into a deep squatting position and then back up. Just watching him, my knees were already hurting. He repeated this 'exercise' for several times.

"I'm 95 years old", he said to me.

"Look what I am still able to do."

He told me he still feels strong and agile, only his eyesight isn't that good.

I got curious and so I asked him why he is in such a good state, according to his opinion.

For a while he didn't say anything. Then, with a grin on his face, he answered, "I have always been in motion. All my life I moved my body a lot. I like it."

This was always the answer I got when talking to elderly fit people. I was always told that they had moved their body a lot and that they still do it.

They mainly went outdoors inhaling fresh air and they enjoy it. After work, which was mostly outdoors too and involved physical labour, they walked through woods and meadows in order to relax and enjoy life. They hadn't felt tired and exhausted back then. Spending spare time in nature would have been recovery enough.

You're not old and frail.
You make yourself old and frail.
Don't slack off, especially when getting along in years.

Once I met an 84 year old woman, wildly gesticulating that she just got back from the beach. She had surfed her first wave ever, lying down on a foam board. She said that she hadn't had so much fun in a long time. I was overwhelmed to see an elderly lady having so much curiosity and zest for life.

Stay always in motion and never stop until you die.
To conclude, essential movements of species appropriate exercising will be pointed out again. I am going to repeat a small selection of natural movements:

Walking
Running
Squatting
Stretching
Pulling
Pushing
Lifting
Pressing
Climbing
Descending
Hanging
Dangling
Jumping
Balancing
Crawling
Stooping


From now on perform these movements regularly, preferably outdoors in nature.
At the beginning, you'll certainly feel a bit stiff.
That'll change quickly.
Just stick to it.


Come on, it's fun!

# III. Species appropriate soul life

Everyday life has an influence on our mental and emotional balance. Most of us live a life they were born and socialized into. This is considered a 'normal' life and we rarely have doubts about it. We usually don't think that this might not be human nature. Sometimes we may feel empty and unfulfilled, wondering about life's essence. Occasionally we may be plagued by fears, but there are plenty of things to distract ourselves.

We stay in relationships and activities, although we can't find any fulfilment. There's just nothing else to do, nothing to hold onto. Some of us might fall into emptiness.

We are longing for a deeper meaning, for support and security.

We suspect there must be 'something', a primal trust, some kind of connection to something 'bigger'.

Most people have lost or simply forgot this kind of connection. It's an access to life's essence, simultaneously leading us to ourselves.

You might be lucky still feeling connected to creation. It's the door to your *self*. It's a deep feeling of security, regardless of time and space. It would be wonderful if you're familiar with it. You're fortunate knowing these kinds of feelings.

Modern ways of life still could have drifted you far away from creation's energy and you're currently not able to feel a connection. You are therefore looking for support and satisfaction in the outside world, rather than finding it within you.

Never forget, just by existing, you're always connected to creation. You're a part of it, as long as you live and beyond.

At this moment you might not be able to access this type of connection. The reasons could lay in the dissimilar lifestyle you're living, being out of joint.

Applying species appropriate eating and exercising into your life can lead you back to connecting, finding this wonderful place within you.

In addition, there are more things to consider.

Let's take a look at it in a practical way.

What is species appropriate soul life about?

## Conscious selection of stimuli and information

Everything we're seeing, hearing, feeling, tasting or smelling, everything we're touching with our senses leaves a trace in us. It has a big influence on our life, even if we're not aware of it. It's not just impressions we absorb with our senses being of considerable importance. We're unconsciously absorbing lots of information we cannot perceive with our senses, taking place on another, an even finer level.

Electrical, radio and satellite waves are just some examples to describe information we neither can see, nor hear, nor touch. They're still around, constantly active. Therefore, they have an effect on us.

The same applies to human beings' thought waves. They are incessantly flowing around us.

Energies of nature, plants and animals, also interact with our system.

Our organism is never independent of its environment. It is rather a part of it. It has to be if it wants to survive. It needs to breathe the air that surrounds it, no matter whether it is clean or dirty.

Receiving stimuli and information brings reactions and consequences. Stimuli and information should therefore be well chosen. We need to ask ourselves the following question:

What type of lifestyle can be considered as species appropriate?

What kind of stimuli would we naturally be exposed to?

Let's take some of our senses.

Let's look at sources of stimuli we're receiving.

Sight: In a natural way of life, we would see trees, flowers, forests and meadows. We would absorb a lot of natural green and look at rivers or lakes. We would be in constant presence of sky and soil, sun, moon and stars. We would see many animals around us.

We wouldn't look at houses, concrete, steel or factories; there wouldn't be any paved roads, traffic lights or lanterns to perceive. Neither would you see cars, televisions or computers. We wouldn't have any advertising around us. There wouldn't be any newspapers and magazines to read. All of this is constantly pouring an overload of unnatural information into our system. Once in us, dissimilar stimuli are taking over, secretly affecting us.

Hearing: We would listen to the wind, the rustling of trees, the ripple of water, to bird's songs and sounds of other creatures surrounding us. Oftentimes we would perceive deep silence, deeply touching and soothing our system.

We wouldn't be surrounded by unnatural noises. We wouldn't be exposed to sirens, cars or drills. We wouldn't hear the sound of televisions, nor radios, nor constant music.

Touch: Your skin would be exposed to sun, wind and rain and not be constricted by clothing and shoes.

You would touch leaves, trees, fruits and of course your fellow people.

Taste and Smell: Imagine now on your own, what would you taste and smell?

It is important to understand that everything you perceive has an effect on your system. We cannot separate body and soul. Our system is internally connected. In the same way, we're interconnected with our supposedly 'external' environment. I therefore repeat: We are one with our environment and not separated from it.

Fellow human beings are also influenced by the world's various stimuli.

Being in exchange with others reinforces our experience of supposed 'reality'. Our world's view becomes a self-sustaining system. Negative, confusing thoughts and emotions of your fellow man are triggered by the same dissimilar lifestyle as your own thoughts and emotions. We might feel dismayed or sad when someone insults us or speaks harshly of us. These are just muddled thoughts meeting other muddled thoughts.

In order to keep 'reality's' formation, we all make sure that in the end, everything remains at status quo. 'Life' takes its usual course and everyone considers it as being 'normal'.

Check and carefully select the stimuli you are receiving.

Start with having your TV turned off, even if it's difficult. Stop reading any kind of newspaper. Believe me; you'll really hear about important events anyway. What do you get when absorbing information of mostly negative events? How does it benefit others if you do not act? If you want to help, then do it. The best place to start is right in front of your doorstep anyway. With silent pity or lust for sensation no one is helped, neither you nor others.

You won't miss anything.

From now on, stop reading magazines. They pretend and flutter around; trying to let you know what is the norm in our world. They have an extensive impact on your subconscious mind in terms of how and what you should be, or how and what you should not be. From now on always use clear thoughts in order to differ between right or wrong. Generally avoid all information not being useful, pulling you away from your path in life. Be alert and on guard of this unnecessary kind of ballast. Of course you can read something once in a while, but be careful what kind of input you are going to get. Read books that are extremely uplifting, books with exceptional wisdom, written by people bringing light and peace into this world.

Whenever possible, keep the radio and computer completely turned off. Both equipment cause a constant overloud of stimuli and information, be it unconsciously.

Listen to music only once in a while. Instead, be fully present when doing it. You'll realize sound can be even more beautiful and uplifting listening consciously. It might touch you on a profound level. If you're not constantly overstimulated, if your receptive system isn't clogged with information, you'll be more sensible and receptive in general.

It's not about banning civilization. The point is to reveal what we actually do to our system and to be aware of it. You can certainly use the good things of modern culture, but be aware that everything you're exposed to has an impact on you.

Keep that in mind and align your life accordingly.

Avoid unnecessary and damaging stimuli in particular.

Initially, you might experience feelings of emptiness or boredom. If that's the case, don't give up.

Continue reducing input of information and regard it as an experiment. After six weeks, take a look and see what has changed. Maybe you'll realize how much you unconsciously crammed your life with stimuli and information out of sheer habit.

What to do with all this stuff?

Is there any space left for new insights?

Is there any room left for your inner being to develop and express itself?

Become empty and let yourself fill with your true nature.

I would like to tell a well-known Zen story I always enjoy reading:

A Japanese master received a professor of philosophy. The Japanese master poured his visitor a cup of tea. When the cup was full, he continued pouring tea in it. The Professor watched the cup overflowing until he could no longer restrain himself: "Stop! The cup is overflowing; there is no space to pour in more."

The Master said: "Like this cup of tea, you are full of your own opinions and brooding. How can I teach you Zen if you have not emptied your cup?"

From now on always focus on something beautiful and natural, no matter where you are.

Imagine you're sitting at a bus stop. You're waiting. What is it you're looking at?

Do you put your gaze on this grey wall to the left or do you set it on the nice tree to your right?

It all starts with a decision from you. You can decide with what kind of sights and sounds you are feeding your soul.

Just deciding to look into another direction as described in this 'waiting for the bus' example, you can make a difference.

We can nourish our soul by focussing on this green tree, observing its leaves, moving in the wind. As you're waiting for the bus to arrive, you automatically get nourished.

Our senses are programmed to perceive specific stimuli we are meant to perceive in order to feel harmonious and complete. Meadows, trees, plants, skies, streams, chirping birds and rustling leaves are the kinds of sensations making us human. We are familiar with them from time immemorial. They are perceptions of pure unadulterated nature without blocks of flats and pylons. They express pure life you can see and feel.

Experiencing this, you get in contact with feelings I call eternity. It is so touching. It is big and yet so close and accessible. You literally get embraced by 'the big' when opening up. If we, however, lack these kinds of impressions, we get torn in our wholeness.

Unfortunately, often-times we do not notice that. Day by day dissimilar stimuli add up until we don't feel well any longer, wondering why. We don't understand it. We get frustrated, blaming our bodies or others.

Usually we are way too busy to be aware of all these processes. We don't notice them. At some point we simply feel exhausted and empty.

Life doesn't need to be that way when being aware of nature's laws.

Every single second of your life you're absorbing all kinds of impressions. Be it sights or sound, you perceive day and night and this has an impact on you, even if you're not aware of it.

I therefore repeat myself once again: consciously drive down your environmental stimuli. You can do it. You just have to decide to take that path. Set priorities. Turn off the radio, even while driving. Put a blanket over your TV and leave it there. Choose in full awareness not to read a single newspaper or magazine anymore.

At first this might bring you boredom. It can even make you feel nervous and unhappy. Just continue and wait to see what is going to happen after doing it for a while. You'll get more in contact with yourself and your life's little truths. Allow it to happen. You'll be rewarded.

Our lives are currently filled with all kinds of artificial sounds and impressions.

We might like them, but often-times they stop us from finding peace, because they're not made of pure life energy – we have created them.

Think of traffic noise, phones' ringing, blocked views of the vast sky in our cities, all this concrete and the colour grey.

Are you not tired of it either?

Constant starring in our computer, surfing the worldwide web, all can steal a lot of precious life energy.

It disturbs our sleep and recovery process to a large extent, even if there are plenty of hours in between.

From now on, try to handle available stimuli with awareness. Avoid unnecessary input. In the long run this will lead you to more well-being and satisfaction.

Don't be fooled by your mind. Be in control of it. You are the master in your house, not your tangled thoughts, desires or lust.

Whether it is leisure activities, sports or just a lunch break at work, it's on you to decide. You have the choice to create your life.

It already starts with changing little things. What are you going to focus on? Will you stare at the grey wall to the left or at the green tree to the right?

Keep in mind that everything we perceive leaves a trace in us. Even perceiving on a subtle level has an effect on you.

## Nourishing Relationships and Community

Other people's thoughts also have an impact on you. They are emitted energy waves, present in the environment.

Don't allow other people to pull you down all the time.

If you're currently sick, this is of utmost importance.

You now need positive life force, not sorrow and hopelessness.

Life is now and there's nothing wrong with it.

Surround yourself with people who are well disposed towards you and others; people who can be happy for you and wish you good. Surround yourself with laughter, peace and merriment. Life is precious. It's too short to walk around grumpy all the

time. What is really that bad with life itself? Is it really worth it to give up your daily joy of life?
In the end we are all going to die anyway. Why should we be in such a hurry to feel dead while we are still alive?

Be vigilant when people constantly run others down, criticizing everything. Surround yourself with good people and good thoughts. Create a loving environment, giving you confidence and security.
Like it is with most primates, survival in nature is best secured when living in a community. We don't feel well spending too much time alone. It is our programming, drawing our attention. We might get alarm signals to finally join a clan or something alike. Thus, nature ensures that we continue to stay alive. It is hard to guess how community life is supposed to look these days. The answer to this question currently can't be given. There are studies showing monkeys having different types of characters, taking on different roles and positions in social structure. Some individuals remain more for themselves; others are very interested in communicating.
Arrange your immediate environment as it is currently best for you. Living in a family, community, in partnership or simply on your own is

not the point. Regardless of living circumstances, it is important to create good and nourishing relationships in your life in whatsoever form.

If you really don't feel like doing something, learn how to say "no". Your health is the most important thing. Others will also benefit in the long run because finally saying "yes" allows you to be authentic and present, attentive to clearly interact and take action.

## Positive thinking and mind control

Disciplining our mind is very important. We are able to reprogram our way of thinking. Our mind has been given to us in order to use it and not it using us. Don't become a slave of circulating and negative thoughts, neither yours nor those of others. They have a big effect on emotions, health and actions.

If negative thoughts come up, say 'stop'.

Instead try to think clearly and positively.

Decide now to do so.

It is up to you.

Don't allow yourself to have too many negative thoughts.

Decide to stop this pattern replacing each negative thought with a positive one. It's a matter of practice; it's about establishing a habit.

Strongly counteract this with the power of positive thoughts and love for creation, including all its beings.

Think positive.

Yes, it is that easy.

Just do it.

I repeat myself: replace each negative thought with a positive one. You have to really want it and then just do it.

Even if you don't believe in positive self-talk, continue doing it.

If certain positive thoughts appear unrealistic to you, do it anyway. Do it consistently.

You will see things change.

You can retrain your brain by creating new habits, practicing daily. It's powerful. After a while, thinking negatively will be a difficult thing to do.

From time to time perform mental exercises. For example, "Today I am not going to deprecate people I meet", or, "Today I will treat myself very caring". There's not much about it and it doesn't take a lot of effort either.

Be 'here and now' and be it more each day. Living species appropriately, being in contact with nature, this happens almost automatically. In addition, you could meditate or learn other techniques to relax. You can find a way to stop constant negative thought patterns and brooding. It's a waste of energy. It doesn't lead you anywhere. If necessary, take time to think about stuff, but do it mindfully. After a while, let the topic move on. Come back to 'here and now'.

Let go and take a look around you. What do you see? What do you hear? What's going on around you, here and now in this moment? Can you hear a bird's song somewhere or rain dripping on your roof? Are there clouds moving in the sky above you?

Go outside into nature. Clear your mind. Consider the saying: "Never trust a thought that is not born in fresh air".

Write down notes with positive words, thoughts or sentences that have a good influence on you.

Set up these notes so you can see them daily.

Practice positive affirmations. Your thoughts are energies, having a big impact on your present and future life.

Read books about this topic.

I repeat: Meditate, learn relaxation techniques and apply them by performing them regularly. Stick to the power of habit.

Remember to breathe evenly.

Breathe.

Don't hold your breath.

Relax your body, hands, face and feet.

Sing, make music. Be creative. Look out for people in order to do it together, be it a choir or other creative groups.

**Less is more**

Each day deliberately set priorities. You can't do everything.

What is really important? How can you keep your inner balance each single day? Every morning make a conscious decision of how you want to perceive and perform your day.

Design your life.

Observe yourself when feeling stressed or worried.

Do you tighten up your muscles?

How about your fingers?

Do you clench your fists?

Are your facial muscles tensed, your eyes, your forehead or your jaw?

What is your breath doing?

Are you still breathing evenly or are you holding your breath?

There are programs within us running automatically. Muscle tension and acceleration of breathing are very well developed methods, helping us to prepare for flight or fight when being at risk. These types of programs were not designed to be constantly active.

The amount of stress and worries we are loading upon us these days is an inappropriate and inhuman behaviour. Of course our organism is reacting.

When do we give our system the signal 'all-clear' so it can relax and recharge its batteries?

Our society is highly ill having exaggerated notions of performance on one hand and excessive hedonism on the other hand.

Generally, the taking of a break in order to rest is often lacking.

'Less' can actually be 'more'. You are more present when doing less. You get much more out of one activity than performing many things in a half-hearted, unconscious way. Reduce your activity list.

Take one day a week in order to do nothing, nothing at all. Lie down and rest. It's not about generally being lazy. It's about moderation. As already mentioned, the level of performance orientation and pleasure seeking society considers being 'normal' is more than too much.

By now, we don't live the life of one person any longer. Instead, most people do so much they live the lives of three people simultaneously.

No wonder so-called stress diseases accumulate in modern world.

You are not a machine.

If you have so much discipline to fulfil all expectations all of the time, then show yourself that you can apply just as much discipline taking breaks and letting things be the way they are, once in a while. You should do that especially when feeling tired or sick.

Don't wreck yourself.

Instead of acting blindly and automatically, take a conscious approach on everyday life.

Think carefully before doing something. Always consider the consequences of your actions.

Ask yourself: Do I really want to do this?

We are our own slaves and we don't even realize it. The bigger your house, the more you have to clean. The more clothing you own, the more you have to think what you want to wear. In his famous book *Walden,* written in the 19th century, the author Henry Thoreau provides us with a wonderful description about these circumstances. Up to these days his observations are of great value. Which of all the things you own do you really need?

Get rid of stuff you don't really use, taking valuable time, energy and living space.

It is very likely that you're surrounded by belongings you don't need at all. What you mostly need, however, is to finally breathe fresh air while listening to the birds.

The current life pace and rapid rhythm of our beloved vibrant civilization isn't quite natural and human either. It simply doesn't meet our natural disposition. These days our pace of life is way too fast. Our inner clock has its very own rhythm, adapted to nature.

To enable healthy processing of stimuli, we need to act on it. We don't feel good in the long run never meeting our system's needs.

We are organisms intended to get around in time and space in a certain way, by walking and running. These days there are many other options available, like airplanes or cars, bringing a fast pace into our life and processing system. How can we deal with all that?

How can we be those blissful beings that we actually are? Look at other organisms. They are so alive, aren't they?

We need to raise our awareness on what is affecting our well-being, installing new strategies and solutions. At least we should open up some space for compensatory activities in daily life. There are plenty of opportunities.

Less is more. You are not missing anything. In your spare time, you don't have to go to three different meetings in order to please everyone or not to miss anything. Shut down your activity level when it's getting dark outside. Slowly and gradually relax and let go of the day's events. Come to rest and remember you're not a machine you can turn on and off by just pushing a button.

Treat yourself consistently in a determined way, yet always gently by loving yourself. Take good care of yourself and keep your boundaries. You can apply both things simultaneously. Remember to encourage yourself rather than demand too much from yourself.


We are way too civilized; we are domesticated. It's important to get things out of our system.

Express yourself. Sing as often as you can. Scream as loud as you want to, right into the forest or while driving your car. Be creative, not giving anything about being 'good' in expressing yourself. Stop worrying about what other people think of your creations. Do handicraft, start to draw, play music. Who cares?! Never forget to laugh either. Your life is short.

**Treating yourself and other living beings with love**

Treat yourself well, lovingly caring of body and soul. Don't blindly follow behaviour and advices of mainstream life.

What is really good for you in the long run?

Stick to a peaceful, quiet life with natural food, lots of exercise and fresh air. Start to live more species appropriately. Mindfully integrate the species appropriate aspects mentioned here. Apply them to your life without undue harshness or criticizing yourself. Just stick to it. Do not confuse gentleness with indifference or neglect. Be determined, yet always affectionate with yourself.

Species appropriate living will reward you with a balanced and peaceful mind. Surround yourself with good things. Nourish mind and body in a positive way.

Each action you're performing is connected to your environment. Each action you are doing has an impact on you.

The origins and energies of the products you use can also influence you.

Where do your products come from?

How did they arise? How are they invented and tested?

In which way do they affect you?

There are many actions we're performing without being aware of consequences. My teacher, Franz Konz, really made me deal with animal testing. He opened my eyes.

I had to shudder deeply and wept bitterly. Each one of us should know what is currently happening behind bars in our beloved 'civilized' world each single day. Everyone needs to know this. Each one of us, even you, has complicity on events ostensibly only for our benefit.

We're all familiar with the term 'animal testing'. The question is, are we aware of the true circumstances? Do we really know the consequences of our own actions?

I don't think so, because otherwise things would be different than they are.

I wasn't aware of it.

In society, truth is often hidden from the crowds. Certain issues are well-kept secrets.

In the following, I would like to show a small fraction of what is going on, what we are all supporting, including you. By purchasing common food, medicine or personal care products, we all choose to support this system.

Change your lifestyle and don't support it anymore. Consider the amounts of suffering you are absorbing just by using these kinds of products. Remember, everything you are in contact with leaves a trace; it has an impact on you.

Don't look away now. Instead watch closely.

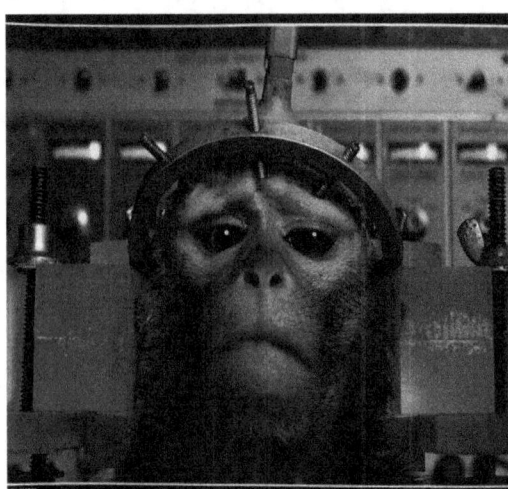

*I just want to cry looking into his eyes.*

Source: AGSTG

Almost everything we're in contact with is tested on animals, be it pharmacology, psychological research, chemical industry, or research on food or weapons.

All of this creates an immense suffering on this planet. It also affects us, our bodies and emotions.

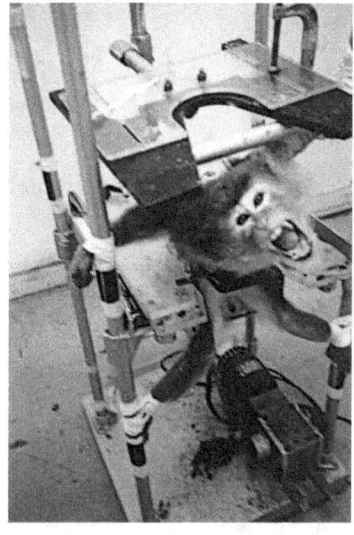

*In the name of science, this creature is going through a lot of suffering.*

Source: AGSTG

In brain research, there are mostly rhesus and cynomolgus monkeys being senselessly tortured, finding a cruel death.

Testing performed on them is extremely painful and absolutely pointless. After a hole got drilled into this monkey's skull, a chamber is installed above it. Electrodes can now directly be inserted into its brain. Most of this is not accessible to the general public.

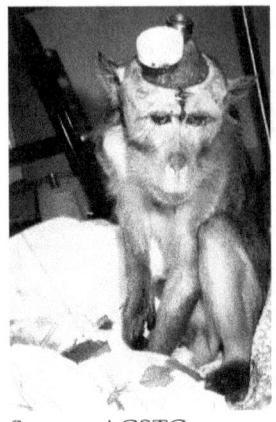

Source: AGSTG

Be it pesticides, herbicides, household products or
toxic gases, everything the researcher's heart desires,
everything that makes our daily life more
comfortable is based on a shuddering and dreadful
background.

Don't get confused now. In research, it's all about
money. It's not about your well-being as science
make you believe.

Research institutions show pictures of healthy test
animals, which supposedly are treated in a caring
way, being well supplied in their laboratories.
Authorities meet the crowds with trivializing
statements like 'an animal experiment is usually just
a small injection'.

Unfortunately reality is shockingly different and everything is therefore done to ensure the public doesn't get to know more.

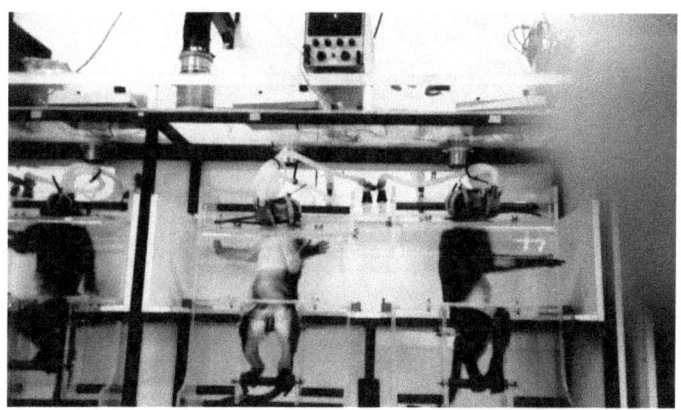

Source: AGSTG

Related documents are barely visible to outsiders, disappearing in official paperwork.
Results of animal studies get published in scientific journals using complicated jargon, keeping it difficult to access for the layman.
Animal research remains secret.

What a price to be paid for our precious ointment.
How many creatures have to suffer for you?

Do you still enjoy buying auspicious creams and pills you only 'need' due to not living species appropriately?

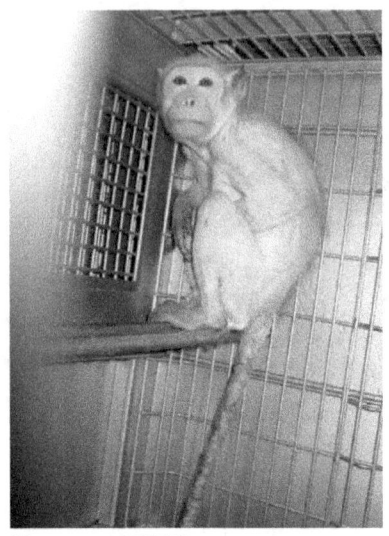

*This poor creature goes through a lot of pain until it finally may die for you.*

Source: AGSTG

Where's the noble person you think you are?
For having the amenities of everyday life, millions of animals are tortured, finding a cruel death. Each chemical material has to be tested in animal experiments. This is even required by law. It doesn't matter whether it is spray paint or shoe polish. Better safe than sorry.

Animal studies aren't limited to mice, rats and monkeys.

Other animals get used by laboratory experiments, like our beloved dogs, cats, rabbits, hamsters or guinea pigs.

Goats, horses, cattle, pigs, chickens, birds, fish, donkeys and dolphins are also caught in this horrible net of researchers' egos.

In publicly accessible media there can't be found any real information about these issues. It is outrageous the way we get lulled and duped in the name of science.

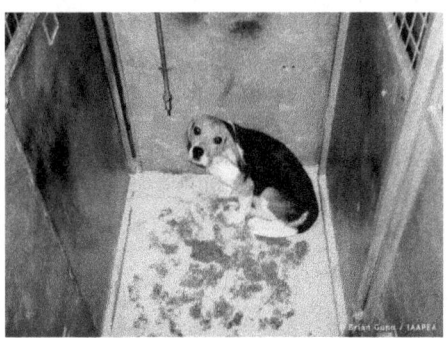

Source: Brian Gunn/IAAPEA

Because of their docility and submissiveness, Beagles are often abused for research purposes. They get picked by big tobacco companies in order to test tobacco products.

The 'right mixture' of any common cigarette is based on cruel animal experiments.

This little guy will soon be taken out of his cage. He will get a hole drilled through his throat.

Then, over a period of several months, concentrated cigarette smoke will be put into his lungs in order to examine long-term effects of smoking.

Rats and mice are also abused for this purpose. Researchers place masks over their head, forcing them to 'smoke' permanently. They are interested in seeing how long animals 'survive' when constantly inhaling this toxic mixture.

Fetuses of pregnant monkeys are poisoned with nicotine to investigate smoking during pregnancy. Then, shortly after being born they get killed in order to examine their lungs.

All this research is complete nonsense.
Please, can't you see that?

If you want to poison yourself then go ahead.
What do innocent animals have to do with it?

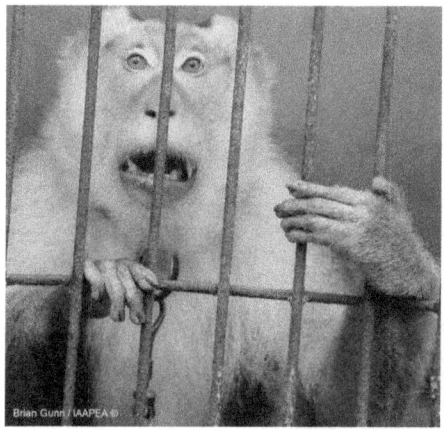

Source: Brian Gunn/IAAPEA

In Europe, about 12 million animals are currently abused in research projects. In the USA, the number of creatures that are suffering every day in order to make our life convenient is even higher; statisticians estimate more than 25 million animals are affected. What a crime we are committing to creation!

This is even a low estimation. In the USA, unfortunately, there are no accurate figures available on how many animals are actually abused because rats, mice and birds are not included in statistics.

They just don't count.

'Only' vertebrate animals like dogs, cats, primates or rabbits are 'worth' being in U.S. statistics, piling up to over a million.

Additives you are using in everyday life are the results of animal experiments too.

Testing the safety of consumer durables often times is mandatory by law.

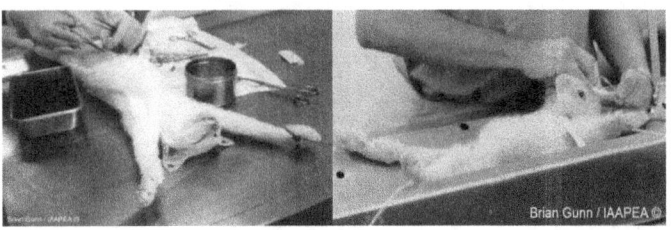

Source: Brian Gunn/IAAPEA
*Do we call our life really harmonious and free of violence? This rabbit didn't even get an aesthetic.*

Why does everything remain in secret?

There's a reason why no one can hear an animal screaming. What is going on behind all this barbed wire of laboratory walls? In order to prevent noise, the animals' vocal cords get severed. No screaming or crying can leave the laboratory. Crime can be simple and easy.

For our vanity, innocent animals also have to suffer. With Botox, you can't just smooth out wrinkles. With only one tablespoon of the active substance botulinum toxin, you can poison a whole lake. Even the smallest production of Botox must therefore be sharply tested, because overdosing the end user would be fatal. Serving this purpose half a million animals are annually facing an excruciatingly death. All this happens out of pure vanity – not wanting any wrinkles.

How do you think your fragrant sunscreen got produced?

Instead, why don't you just go into the shade?

Maybe next time…?

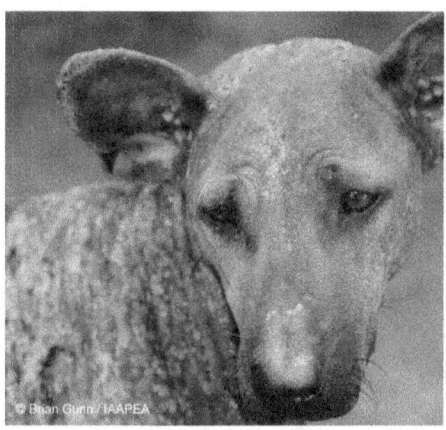

*Another victim…*

Source: Brian Gunn/IAAPEA

Medical research is highly praised.

If we'd just know what it's about, the things we're supporting, that we highly admire. If we'd just know what it really involves. I wish we'd be aware of it.

Despite all efforts, money and the deaths of millions of animals, people still die of cancer. How to do research on this type of disease? In order to 'fight' it, one first needs to have an organism with cancer to experiment with. For research purposes innocent healthy creatures get therefore poisoned until they finally develop a malignant tumour.

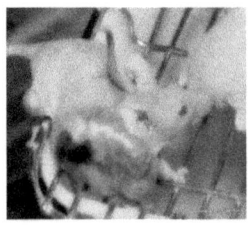

*Induced tumour formation in cancer research*

Source: Brian Gunn/IAAPEA

After researchers achieved what they wanted, the poor creature then was subject to cancer tests, before finally ending up in the trashcan. I guess the experiment wasn't successful.

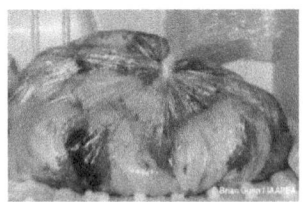

*Look very closely…*

Source: Brian Gunn/IAAPEA

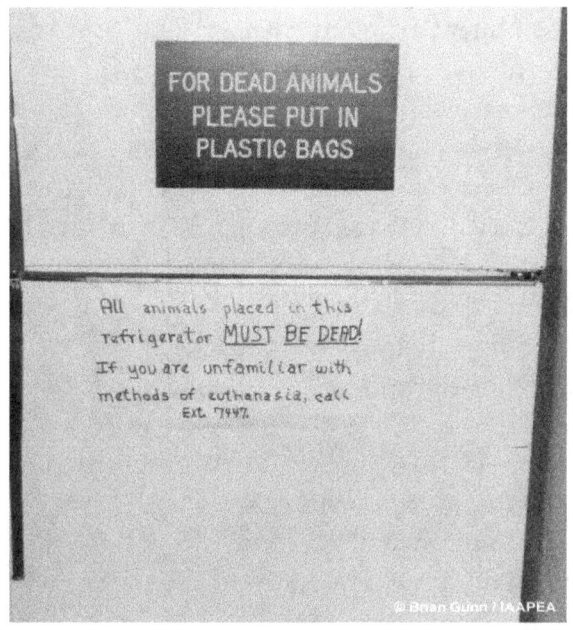

Source: Brian Gunn/IAAPEA
*Sometimes the poor creatures are not even given the mercy of death.*

Atrocities like this are not confined to brain experiments or cancer research. They are also very common in other areas of medical research.

Think logically. Ask yourself how an ointment for severe burning is invented. How did it get tested? Of course, a creature has to be burned first in order to test the ointment's ingredients. Imagine on your own, how this example continues.

I repeat: In order to authorize drugs and medication, animal testing is required by law. Let's take another example. How can stomach remedies be tested without having a damaged stomach being available? Prior to experimenting, researchers pump lots of acid into an animal's stomach. Again I will leave it to your imagination how that would look like.

Do you really think these creatures don't feel any pain?

Vaccinations, artificial joints and bypass surgeries are also procedures tested on animals.

Who do we think we are?

How can we think we don't have to pay the price for the suffering we're causing?

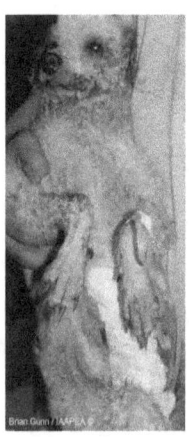 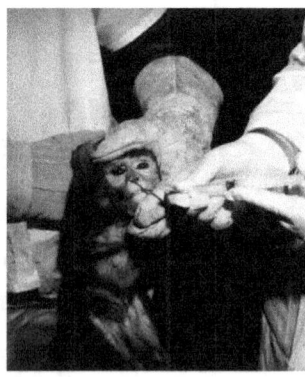

Source:
Brian Gunn/
IAAPEA

Most animal experiments are pointless anyway. Often times results are not transferable to humans and developed products are causing damage to us in the long run. We are abusing innocent creatures just because we're too comfortable to live in a more species appropriate way.

I don't even want to mention the practice of so-called basic research. It's about pure satisfaction of scientific curiosity. The point of interest is floating. Respective researchers are simply looking for answers to the following question: "What if…?"

Now you have more of an idea of what is going on at the expense of innocent creatures, thanks to taxes and well intentioned donations.

Cruelties also take place in research projects that don't even focus on substances. Animal testing is highly practiced in psychological research projects asking the same question: "What happens if…?"

There are thousands of experiments serving 'our important science'.

One of them is analysing social behaviour of a disabled organism. What happens if you paralyze both hind legs of a cat? How does it affect its social behaviour? Researches are also interested in observing a cat's behaviour that is forced to wear a mask since birth in order to remain blind.

'Scientists' then are able to investigate 'social' consequences.


Let's be serious now.

Let's think with a clear mind.

Is all that really necessary?

Wake up and bring this madness to an end. Stay away from all these products. Instead help yourself whenever possible.

You now know what is going on under lock and key, even in your environment.

Modern countries like the USA or Germany have huge experimental laboratories.

From now on, you're in charge by taking conscious decisions in favour or against these conditions because you're aware of the situation. You know what is going on.

You know what it's about. You can tell the story behind each pill and tablet you are ingesting as well as with every ointment or chemical product you're using.

Torturing other living beings, no matter if consciously or unconsciously is such a negative energy. It's absolutely dissimilar to our nature. We're therefore tormenting ourselves.

Are you really happy?

Don't forget we're connected with everything around us. We are not separate organisms. You can personally bring these cruelties to an end, finding health yourself.

I know this part of the book isn't easy to swallow, but no one is helped lacking awareness. It wouldn't help you. This chapter is about species appropriate soul life.

Harmonious and peaceful interactions with yourself and other living beings you are sharing space with on this planet has a profound impact on your health. Therefore circumstances cannot continue to exist if you want to be healthy. Stay away from these products so that at least you'll absorb a bit less suffering. You'll feel the difference.

### Realistic dealing with life and death

Each day you get to breathe. Each day you get to experience is a very precious gift.

Are you aware that your life can end here and now in each single moment? Really?

Most of the time, we don't have this awareness. We make our lives difficult, feeling irritated by minor and trivial incidents.

Once, on a small island, an old lady said to me, "Modern people just don't know that they will die." Physical death is present in every single second, always and everywhere. Keep that in mind. To practice your memory, several times a day try to imagine 'death' sitting right on your shoulder. It is present and close. It is a part of you. It is your destiny for this lifetime.

Thanks to my friend Linda, there's another beautiful metaphor:

Imagine standing on the edge of a very high cliff, the raging wide ocean below.

How does life function? Staying within this metaphor, at the beginning of our life, we are on top of the cliff and jump down. The free fall is our life. From the moment of jumping down, which is the beginning of our life, we are automatically determined to die, ending up in the wide ocean below.

Some people might hit a ledge and therefore die a few seconds earlier. Others fall all the way down without hitting the cliff at all, but everyone gets to the bottom and ends up being dead. From the very moment we're born, we are jumping towards death. In everyday life, we are rarely aware of this fact.

Rather than wavering with trifles as if they're the world's most important issues, visualize yourself being in free fall, arguing with the person next to you, also being in free fall. It's such a hilarious picture to imagine. Arguing in this situation seems absolutely pointless, doesn't it?

Death is always there. It is always close to you.

Listen to it every single day. Don't devalue it.

Remember and accept the fact that you can die at any moment, whether it happens at home or in the car. You can always die, no matter how many safety precautions you're taking. You're not in control.

Keeping this in mind, you'll live your life differently. What is really important? Are things really that terrible?

Do we really have to take everything so seriously?

Think about it next time, when you get upset about something, feeling caught up in your problems.


In modern society death is locked away. It is ignored and seen as something bad, something that is very sad.

Yet, it's a natural event and part of life.

Without death there's no life.

If your cells wouldn't die, your body couldn't create new ones.

If that would be the case, you would have ceased to live a long time ago.

What a pity that death is related to so much fear and sadness. It would be good to get in contact with death, seeing dead bodies while being young.

We then could learn that dying is part of life, a natural process and nothing to fear.

Luckily there are still cultures approaching death in different ways. In some countries people naturally die at home. The person's dead body stays three days within the family home before being buried so that the soul can let go. Relatives and friends are also able to say goodbye. All children have access to the dead one too. It is something 'normal'.

In other societies, the bodies of the dead are publicly burned. Confronting this, a western person can only remain with the following aphorism, "Cremation is education". We literally get to see then that our body is impermanent.

Life implies constant change.

Going into nature, it's easy to observe this in a practical way. You constantly see organisms dying and new ones emerging.

Dealing with death might be difficult for us because we still believe we are not a part of nature. Instead we think we have a special role in creation. We might not want to realize that we simply can't control life's laws. Life and death is a dance. It's the rhythm of life. It's a game with life energy.

I do admit this chapter wasn't an easy one either.
Let the information now sink deeper into your system. The level of species appropriate soul life is very diverse. All its aspects are as important for your healing as all the other parts previously revealed in this book. Let's take a brief review. What was this level about?
Consider the following aspects:

- Conscious selection of stimuli and Information
- Nourishing relationships and community
- Positive thinking and mind control
- Less is more
- Treating yourself and other living beings with love
- Realistic dealing with life and death

Don't be afraid of the changes to happen. Things you previously valued a lot might be put into perspective, might be modified.
You will feel that life is flow.

Things are emerging and disappearing.

It is a constant renewal.

Everything functions harmoniously, following an inherent rhythm.

You will realize that you're safe in creation.

You are therefore ready to let go if necessary.

I will now tell you a little bit more about the experiences I had, integrating this level into my life.

*As usual, I went to the urban forest in order to inhale fresh air and do my regular workout in nature.*

*As I was walking through the forest I grabbed a whole bunch of leaves, inhaling their smell.*

*I was watching the birds, carefully listening to their songs.*

*I leaned on a tree, looking up into its branches.*

*Finally, I stepped into a small meadow, a beautiful spot to start my workout.*

*At first I looked to the right.*

*I realized I was gazing at utility poles and house cusps protruding through the trees. I turned to the left and the only thing I got to see was sky with clouds passing by. It was that easy. I wanted to feed my mind with positive impression. I therefore decided quite consciously to look at trees and open skies while doing my workout. For the next hour I wanted to watch birds and clouds moving along while exercising.*

*In full awareness, I decided to change my viewpoint in order to absorb all these movements of pure life energy.*

*I therefore turned my body to the left and set myself accordingly, so that I'd just see nature and no electricity poles or houses. In that moment I wasn't able to change the fact of living in a city, but I could decide about perceiving this very moment. I was able to choose another direction, to get another viewpoint. As a consequence, I absorbed positive and calming stimuli.*

*During my workout, I watched the trees and I became absorbed by the movement of leaves in the wind. I kept my eyes on the purity of lush green nature for a long time. This was also a form of exercising: practicing to focus the mind. I knew everything my system was absorbing had an impact on me. All activities I was performing, everything I perceived with my senses, totalled at the end of the day. It had an influence on my well-being and sleeping quality.*

*For a certain time, I was extensively engaged in watching and learning about the variety of plants. For quite a while I closely looked at leaves and flowers in a precise manner. One night I went to bed and closed my eyes. In that moment I started to get visions in front of my inner eye. All I was seeing were the bright beautiful flowers I observed during the day. I had totally absorbed them into my system. Remembering these beautiful images, I fell into a restful sleep.*

Day by day I became more aware of this planet's beauty. I felt I finally got back a clear vision. I saw it as a consequence of performing a species appropriate lifestyle in general.

It was overwhelming having this sudden view of immense beauty around me.

Coincided with feeling embraced and secure in creation, I too began to accept myself. I realized love and acceptance for other fellow humans also had expanded. In every person I wanted to see my brother and sister. Didn't we all inherit the same power of creation?

From now on, I wanted to take better care of myself. Only if I was ok, I could bring happiness to others. The way to contentment couldn't pass my own self.

I wrote memos with positive affirmations. I placed them visible to me whenever possible. I specifically trained my mind.

This also included less contact with people constantly thinking negatively. I was instead looking for interactions with more positive thinking people in general so that I could reprogram my view on life. I knew I had to retrain my mind in order to be healthy. I had to learn to say "no". Yet, I didn't want to hurt anyone. I wanted to stay open for people around me needing help, consolation or advice. I understood I could still do this, but not if it would harm *myself. Things needed to be in moderation according to personal limits, which are always temporary.*

*Positive thinking was a new thing to me. It was therefore quite fragile. Wanting to expand and integrate it into my life, I had to take good care of myself, especially in the beginning. I didn't want to fall back into old thought patterns; instead I was willing to consider all aspects of life as positive ones.*

*I also trained my brain to be a bit creative. I started to draw and make music. I wasn't familiar with being an artist, yet I knew in recent decades my brain had been working fairly one-sided. It was well trained in mental activities such as intellectual or rational thinking.*

*I really wanted to activate other parts of my brain however. I started colouring images like a little child because I didn't have the confidence to draw.*

*I also started drumming and singing in a group. Initially, I had to push myself so that I'd really go and do it. These days I feel much more balanced using my brain for more than just for rational thinking. I feel more holistic.*

These are just a few impressions. You will have wonderful experiences yourself.

Remember the facilities that are given to you by creation. Now go ahead. Take a life path corresponding to yourself, to your species.

You'll feel much better every day.

I promise you will find many benefits.

Life is so beautiful. You don't want to miss that.

From taking this path you will get so much clarity. Your life's insights will be revealed. You are going to meet the love of creation.

What are you waiting for?

Go and set off.

# IV. Species appropriate habitat

The last level I would like to point out is creating a more species appropriate habitat. There are a few things to mention. If you agree, you can integrate them into daily life, designing your existence accordingly.

It's important to reiterate the value of connecting with natural forces.
'Feel' nature as often as possible. It is made of pure life energy. Go outdoors and listen to the silence, to the tranquillity you can find in it. Spend lots of time inhaling fresh air. Your system needs oxygen. It needs a lot of it, especially when living in civilization. Unfortunately, each day we're exposed to radiation and pollutants. Think about everything we're surrounded with. What are closets and carpets at home made of? Keep in mind the mattress you sleep on, the clothes you wear or the paint on your walls. A variety of devices are also constantly present. Be it phone, television, computer, printer or refrigerator, everything is ready to operate. Consider all these radio and satellite waves in our atmosphere. They literally beam through your house to your neighbour and so on. Everyone can use them. You can't see

these waves, but it's obvious they are there; otherwise your devices wouldn't work. Take a close look at your place. What do you surround yourself with? At home, too, try to make some changes.

If there's really no way to set your place up in a different manner, going outdoors and spending time in pure nature seems to be the most simple way to recharge and strengthen your system. One day you might live in a more natural environment if you wish so.

*Writing this, I remember being in Central America.*
*I enjoyed being friends with the locals.*
*One of them had a great place in the middle of the jungle. He was an elderly man, very much connected to nature. He had a nice bed, but he had put it outside! He said to me, he needed to sleep under open sky.*
*This man was very sensitive to the life energy surrounding him, even though in an unconscious, more intuitive way. By being in contact with creation's energies he was scooping strength, security and health.*
*There was another senior villager I liked talking to. During our conversation I found out that this old gentleman hiked cross country through the jungle. Shockingly, there were no trails available to use. He just ran through the bushes up and down in deep tropical*

*forest out of pure pleasure, in order to maintain inner peace and well-being. At night he would even sleep in the woods. "But where exactly do you sleep?" I asked. He answered, "I just put a plastic bag on the ground, that's the only thing I take with me."*

*Finally I met a calm forest worker. I asked him if he wouldn't feel lonely, if it wasn't dangerous to work in the jungle all by himself. "Yes, it is a bit dangerous, but here I'm one with God ", he said.*

*Working in the rain forest, he would feel 'Him', feel connected. "I feel happy", he said. He couldn't be in the village all the time, especially not in pubs where, according to his view, people would talk too much nonsense and get drunk. It would bother him, disturbing his feelings of essence and spirit.*

You don't need to live like these interesting contemporaries do.

Nevertheless, consider the impact of pure life force on your system. You are nature. Don't neglect yourself. Stay in contact with the vital forces inside and around you, every single day.

Interestingly we're able to acknowledge our beloved pets' need to live according to their species. We often criticize, "How bad to keep huge dogs in small city apartments. An animal of this size needs to spend its time outdoors, playing and running around. It needs space to move. It will suffer if kept in a small city apartment."

It's funny to hear stuff like that. What about us? Are we really that different? Doesn't our system suffer in a very similar way, spending too much time indoors, not getting enough time to run out?

Who are you and how are you determined to live?

I remember reading an interesting statement: "Living a life that is not appropriate to our species is to us like a fish constantly trying to climb up a tree."

The fish will never be successful, no matter how hard it tries. It would harm itself. Would it continue trying to climb up the tree or not rather go back and swim in the water?

We keep trying.

Isn't that insane?


Look at your daily schedule. Ask yourself, "When do I have time to go into nature?"

Your life is so packed; you probably don't know what to do.

Set up priorities. Create more space.

In order to establish something new, you must dismiss other things first. The day has only 24 hours and you simply can't do everything.

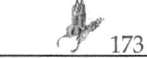 

Be truthful with yourself. You can't do it all at once. What is really important in the long run?

Don't neglect health and well-being for other, far more temporary things.

How does your spare time look like?

Are you really aware of what you're doing in your free time?

Do you feel good about it?

How about afterwards?

From now on, create room for your own healing and well-being. You will easily find more time by no longer watching television. Radically reduce internet 'consumption' down to maybe two hours per week. Stop reading newspapers and magazines. Use new-found time for going outdoors and consciously perceiving nature, even if it is just a park or city forest. You can find pure life force anywhere. Surrounded by concrete, there's always some kind of plant to be discovered. Life energy is unstoppable. I repeat: Spend time outdoors as much as possible.

Do your workout in nature. Persuade friends to meet for a walk instead of sitting in a cafe.

From now on, avoid using chemical products whenever possible. Ask yourself, "Why do I need so many care products, like creams and make-up?"

"Why are body and soul so much out of balance that I can't live without these products?"

From now on, cease to use chemical toiletries. Think of all the harmful substances you're absorbing. Check out components of soap, toothpaste, deodorant, shampoo and moisturizer. Your skin is not made of plastic. It is alive. It is your largest organ. It's excreting substances and also absorbing environmental elements to a large extent. Products you're using don't remain on your skin. They get into your entire system's circulation. Remove lipsticks, balms and promising ointments from your life. You know where these products come from. It is pure chemical industry submerging into your system. I as well, stopped using common soap. I even ceased using conventional shower gel and shampoo. No, I didn't start to stink; neither did I get any lice. I just use water instead. In order to wash my hair I apply lava clay called "Rhassoul" or "Ghassoul" clay. You just mix a few tablespoons of clay with water until a thick paste is formed and use it instead of shampoo. After a few applications you will like it. Skin and hair feel wonderful. It's very simple.

Cease to use deodorant and perfume. Both are pure artificial chemicals. It might be hard to imagine, but you'll no longer need those kinds of things. Before I changed my lifestyle I was sweating a lot. Living a species appropriate life, which includes omitting salt, excessive sweating, belonged to the past.

Believe me, you'll sweat less and you'll have a more pleasant smell in general.

Bring your system back to balance and you no longer need all these products. Don't destroy your natural skin's film by using chemical toiletries.

If you can't live without moisturizer and your skin feels dry, take organic olive oil or organic coconut oil instead.

Keep in mind the water's origin you're using.

Do you have access to natural water?

Think of all the additives, the chlorine in our water system, possibly irritating your skin.

Taking hot showers, using hot water in general, dries your skin out immensely.

From now on abandon using hot water.

Your skin problems will be resolved. Take cold showers only. It's good for you. It makes you tolerate a wide range of temperatures and strengthens your immune system (cf. Galina Schatalova). Living in modern society has made us weak.

Putting things into practice, it's good to take small steps and slowly get familiar using cold water.

*When I finally decided to go with cold water, it was very difficult to get used to. I thought my heart would stop beating. I needed to find a more gentle approach and so, every time I took a shower, it was 'less warm'. I continued lowering the water temperature each time I showered. These days I love to shower cold. I feel good.*

*I feel fresh and clear.*

*Using hot water really dries out my skin. Every time I do it I have this kind of result. Taking hot showers makes me feel weak and tired.*

*In general, I feel less cold. I am much better prepared for a wide range of temperature. Before, I became chill easily.*

*Once I read about Chile's native inhabitants. Several centuries ago, when Spanish people arrived, they noted the following: Wrapped in warm clothes they were sitting around a fire in order to warm up.*

*Indigenous people, hardly wearing anything, were standing at a good distance from the fire and sweat was running down on them because of the heat they felt.*

Exposing our system, our naked skin, to fresh air and sunshine is essential.

This importance includes the whole body, preferably without clothes. We can still respect current morals and customs, but places exist where naked sunbathing is possible. You'll find a spot.

We need to keep in mind unknown consequences of the altered atmosphere. These days, people fear the sunlight. Nevertheless remember that exposing your entire system to light and air on a regular basis is highly important. Watch out using conventional sunscreen. It is composed of carcinogens. Take a closer look.

Your skin is an organ and not the wall of some house you can paint.

Of course you shouldn't suffer from sunburn. Take a slow and gentle approach. Avoid direct sunlight over a long period of time.

If you're going to be in the sun for a while, wear a hat. Even animals look for shade. Most time they spend protected in a thicket of leaves.

Sunlight is very important for you, therefore find a reasonable measurement. Cover yourself with a towel. Go into the shade if you had too much sun or your skin starts to burn. The more you're outdoors, the more your system will get used to it. Changing your diet will also help because 'life' food components make your system tolerate the sun much better. Use sunscreen only if really necessary. You can find less chemical ones in health food stores.

Remember our relatives, the big apes.

They mainly live deep within the forest.

They spend their time both in sun and shade.

Try to swallow fewer pills. Ask yourself, "What kind of a life am I currently living, such that it can only be tolerated by taking pills every day?"

Make changes in your life or in the way you perceive it.

Live with clear senses.

You don't have to suffer. You now have plenty of information on how to implement this.

If you have any doubts whether something's good or healthy for you, just think logically:

"Is it something natural I am going to do or is it not?"

"What if there's no civilization as we know it?"

"How would I act?"

If you don't feel well, then honestly ask yourself:

"What kind of unnatural behaviour did I recently perform?"

You'll quickly recognize causes for not feeling well. You'll know what to change in order to feel better, rather than being helpless about feelings of discomfort.

Let's have a look at your household.

What kind of cleaning products do you use?

How do you wash your clothes?

Are you using chemicals?

By just living your 'regular' life, you are absorbing harmful substances.

Late at night you lie down on a polluted mattress and cuddle yourself into fragrant pillows, breathing in pure chemical detergent and a few fumes of your room's toxic furniture.

At least you should open some windows, don't you think so?

Don't worry; you don't need to be stinky and messy. I am also wearing clothes. I wash them too, with soap nuts. Soap nuts are part of a plant that grows in warmer climates. They are a great detergent. For years I've been using them now and so far I haven't encountered any problems. I even feel better.

How about all the chemical dish detergents you're using?

Fortunately, eating raw and fresh, one doesn't have to wash many dishes. Just rinse off your plates with water. If you really need some soap to clean, get a less aggressive detergent at your local health food store. It might be more expensive, but keep in mind that you're absorbing harmful substances otherwise.

You'll need less soap anyway.

Observe what you're automatically doing throughout the day. Most of the time, we blindly follow society's guidelines without ever questioning them. We are taking over everything that has made us believe, be it out of fear or pure habit. Instead of living other people's concepts, scrutinize everything you're doing and thinking. Advices of so-called 'smart people' in particular, need to be handled with distance. Always remain on a natural path. It is mostly the more easy and simple one.

Take caution. Don't surround yourself with too many electronic devices. Avoid anything artificial if possible. Abstain from air conditioning; stay away from chlorine. Don't use swimming pools or Jacuzzis due this poison's presence.

As already stated, in natural life one thing is connected to the other. It is interdependent, forming a perfect world, exactly done by creation.

Living a pure and healthy lifestyle automatically leads to a pure and healthy planet. There is no unnecessary littering and poisoning. You also put fewer burdens on our planet Earth by abstaining from chemical pollutants. You'll produce less waste in general. There's hardly any chemical waste like plastic. Substances ending up in our precious water are less harmful when living naturally. Rivers and oceans get less polluted; at least you aren't using any chemicals for dishes and clothes.

Don't forget that we are part of the chain. Rivers and oceans will become clouds, raining down on us. In order to live, you need the following: Clean air, healthy soil and good water. It's about essentials, about what your physical life depends on, your health and well-being.

Realize you're not a separate organism; you're in association with all that is. You're a part of it, a small part of the great puzzle, being connected to everything. Now that you have gotten to know the keys of living species appropriately, it is up to you to put things into action. Take your time, do one thing after the other. Realizing your health is increasing, make sure to continue.

*When a year had passed I took stock. What had happened? What had changed?*
*I didn't take any more medicine. I was less susceptible to diseases. I was able to move my body again. I started to exercise. I finally got to sleep. I was positive and filled with an upbeat tune.*

Describing a species appropriate lifestyle is hereby completed for the most part. In the remaining there are a few more topics to be discussed, helpful tools on your path to health and well-being.

# 5. Excursus: Inner Cleansing

Throughout your life, you ingested many things your body wasn't programmed for, be it through diet or medical interventions such as tablets, injections or infusions. Your system is constantly absorbing harmful substances out of your environment. The water you're drinking, air pollution and chemicals in body care products, are impure to you.

Quite a bit has accumulated in your system. This might be harmful in the long run. You are constantly carrying this stuff within you. How can your soul live and thrive? How can you achieve clarity and well-being? How can you have positive thoughts under such conditions?

Our system doesn't know what to do with this alien stuff. For the most part, foreign substances are stored. In some cases this takes place in fatty tissue and blood vessels, otherwise muscle tissue and joints are affected.

Some people have trouble with their stomach and intestines too, getting easily irritated by eating whatever, even fruit.

The reason lies in the intestinal flora's composition. Due to having a dissimilar lifestyle your intestinal flora is less intact. Your system suffers, having temporary disorders.

Don't be startled if you're currently not able to digest properly. Applying a new way of life, your system will recover with time. It will provide space for symbiotic relationships with necessary micro-organisms, which you automatically ingest by eating species appropriately.

In order to be truly successful, internal cleansing is a key. Especially at the beginning it is an important step to clean up your inner body, or better said, "To make it clean it itself up".

Inner cleansing described here in this book is about fasting and colon cleansing.

Both may require some practice and discipline, but you'll feel the benefits.

**Fasting**

Your body is busy with digesting most of the time. Just imagine what you're eating throughout the day. Everything has to be processed down to the smallest detail. This means a tremendous amount of work. Fasting allows your system to take a break. 'Unemployed' body cells have more time now and start to take a look around. They begin to process other things they can find in the system. They can't help it. It's their program. They clean up. You begin to detoxify.

In order to perform a period of fasting, it's better to have some time off. Take some vacation and stay on your own if possible. While fasting, don't expose yourself to excessive stimuli; in particular avoid negative input. You'll be more sensitive, more receptive. Use this state of being and benefit from it. Why don't you wait, observing what is happening during the fast? You might get to know yourself better. Don't watch television, turn off your computer and switch your phone off if possible. Take full advantage of the fast to really fall back on you. Don't allow excessive information, noise and alleged dramas to interfere with your journey to serenity.

While fasting, do an enema every few days. I'll talk more about this shortly. One or two days before starting a longer fasting period, eat a little bit less so that your system can slowly glide into it. After finishing fasting, you should also take it easy. You'll need a few days until you can eat again. Gradually increase your intake of food, of course sticking to a species appropriate diet. Initially just eat a piece of fruit and after a while get some more; otherwise you and your stomach won't feel that well. Your digestive system needs to wake up again and get in motion.

During fasting always stay physically active, as much as you can. Don't lie in bed, even if you totally feel like it. This is very important.

While fasting, ingest only water if possible. This means you won't eat anything at all or drink anything other than non-carbonated water. In the morning you can detoxify with a teaspoon of healing clay, but that's all you should consume. Drink water whenever you're thirsty. Your system might get flooded with toxins from each of your cells. Move your body as much as possible in order to carry out these toxins. You also have to stay in motion, so that your circuit remains stable. Give it a shot.

Never fast if you're on medication. Imagine its impact on your otherwise 'empty' body. If the pill is the only thing your system is ingesting, it will affect you like a huge dose of poison and thus wreak havoc. Don't consume salt either, under any circumstances. Have faith in yourself and remember your body can certainly live a while without eating.

Do a fasting period once or twice a year in order to get a good cleansing. You also clean your house from time to time, don't you? The fasting's duration should depend on how lean you are. If you're very thin, it's sufficient to fast three to five days. If you're of bigger constitution, you could fast for quite a while.

Start to establish one day of fasting per week. This is a very common practice in natural medicine. It is very restoring and relaxing.

All the things we're eating and especially the amount of it isn't really that natural.

Creation is kind and loving. It has so much to give. Constantly having food available to eat whatever we want, whenever we want and how much we want is unnatural. We are overtaxing our system by eating too much food all the time. Our poor system constantly has to work, not getting anything done. Nature is set up in a special way. Food is not always present in absolute abundance. It doesn't kill you. In fact, by taking a break of eating, our body begins to make better use of the food being supplied. One fasting day per week, would that really hurt? It's easy. It's merely 24 hours. You could stop eating Monday at noon and start eating Tuesday around lunchtime. After a few weeks of practice, you'll see how relaxing it is. You will no longer have to deal with unnecessary thoughts and all of the sudden you will have so much time.

Isn't it interesting that fasting is taught by all religions since time immemorial? In so many ways people rely on religion for its morality and doctrine, but when it comes to fasting the Holy Scriptures often tend to be closed.

This book is not about a particular religion; it's about your health. Try to fast and let it surprise you. It has a positive effect on your health. Furthermore, you are going to experience being internally pure. If you become empty, creation, its simple clarity and wisdom, is able to flow through you.

You'll get in touch with your life's essentials, with the core of being. You might sense what creation is made of. It is love, at least according to my experience.

**Colon Cleansing**

We're now going to briefly discuss the topic of colon cleansing. The whole thing sounds a bit ugly and therefore I promise not to go into too much detail.

The simplest way to give your intestines a good cleansing is the so-called hydro-colon therapy. It requires a special device as well as professional handling by a medical practitioner or naturopath. This type of procedure might be practiced in your area. If there are options to choose from, compare different offers. If you can afford it, take a few sessions, like once a week for six weeks in a row.

You can also stay independent, giving yourself an enema, which is cheaper, but not as thorough.

Relax, there is really nothing bad about it.

At your local pharmacy you can buy an enema device, a hose attached to a simple plastic container. You just fill the container with healthy water and put it on a shelf. You kneel or lie down and let the water run into your posterior. It's good to wait for a while, if possible. You will automatically know what's going to be the next step.

It's therefore recommendable to stay in the bathroom while waiting in order to use it right away when time has come.

With a little practice and routine, it's a quick and easy procedure.

At the beginning you can do a small cleansing phase, performing enemas more often, for example once a week. Later on you can fall back on it from time to time.

In the following I'll tell you about my personal experience with inner cleansing. Don't worry; I won't go into deep details here either.

At the same time I started to change my diet, I went to a hydro-colonic treatments clinic once a week. I do admit, at first the whole thing felt very uncomfortable to me.

Again, I thought to myself, "What the heck, the leopard can change its spots."

I went to all of my appointments over a period of six weeks. After a short while I felt very good about it.

Fasting, on the other hand, was not that simple. I decided to do a fast, but showing action was another thing. Somehow there were always more important things happening. Finally I took a calendar. I marked ten days of the following month with no other 'important' events. I decided to keep those days clear. It should appear like being on vacation. I planned the fast like an incoming event and mentally prepared myself. I told everyone about it, so it became even more real. I gathered information about fasting in order to feel more secure and started to practice how to do an enema. When the time had arrived, I bought sufficient amount of spring water. Once again I told my friends that I was going to fast soon and I asked them for understanding and acceptance. I wouldn't be available. I reassured friends and family that I would keep them up to date about my well-being. I was handling the situation in a firm and determined way. Two days before entering the fasting period I already started to eat less. I also made sure to move my body a lot. Then I ate nothing except a *teaspoon of healing clay in the morning. I only drank water.*

*I felt weird. I wasn't sure what to think and if I would like it. Sometimes I felt fantastic, sometimes I felt miserable. Often times I was about to cancel the whole thing. I remembered, however, that I had taken many pills and injections in my life. I wanted to help my body to detoxify. It was too obvious. My system was already getting rid of stuff. It was amazing to see and yet not always a pleasant experience. Strange odours were pouring out from every skin pore. I got bad headaches and felt nauseous.*

*By reading literature on fasting I was able to see these kinds of symptoms as signs of detoxification. They were not characteristics of fasting per se.*

*That gave me hope.*

*I was aware that if I threw up, I'd need to cancel the fast. Luckily this didn't happen and so I kept going. I knew I had to keep my body in motion in order to improve my symptoms, for it was the best method to get rid of overflowing pollutants. I so much wanted to stay in bed instead. I felt bad. I asked a few friends, people who had done fasting before. None of them remembered having such extreme symptoms. I realized I was just strongly detoxifying and my conditions eventually would improve. I had confidence in my body and faith in creation. I held out during some difficult moments and decided to* continue the fast, even though all my friends were shaking their heads. I had already gotten used to that anyway. Once again, I said to myself, "What the heck..." I had nothing to lose. I had been through far worse stages in my life and this time I was at least in some kind of control of what I was doing. I had made a conscious decision and I was always able to cancel it if I wanted to.

During fasting, time was passing by very slowly. Day by day I found more clarity. It was inconceivable. I thought less and started to feel more. My life appeared more transparent. Things got obvious. I started to understand a bit more.

I was cleaning up, inside and outside. I expressed my view on things by directly saying what seemed important to me. I felt so much love.

I began to treat myself mindfully, with lots of care. I had never felt so much love for me and my body. As I went out into nature, I was delighted about everything I perceived, about birds in the sky and the smiling faces of children.

As bad as my body was feeling in between, my feelings, my thoughts, my heart and my soul were clear and pure. I felt glad and grateful.

I felt what I really wanted, what needed to be changed. I sensed being more in contact with myself, being less influenced and distracted. I wasn't 'fed' by other things. I was empty instead, able to receive.

*I needed little sleep; my pulse was slow and even. I was breathing continuously in a deep abdominal way.*

*After seven days of just drinking water, I decided to stop because I had lost plenty of weight. It was time to get back to eating again. Instead of causing damage to myself, I wanted to benefit from what I was doing. It was time. I slowly started to consume some fruit and gradually went back to a species appropriate diet. I felt very hungry. My body wanted to be rebuilt. Unfortunately, I couldn't eat that much. My digestive system had adapted to fasting mode. After a few days it got better. I was gradually able to consume more food. Everything was good. With the resumption of eating, I observed that my thought activity was increasing, feeling a bit less clear. Nevertheless, I felt quite good, probably because of eating fresh and raw food.*

*I never forgot the experiences and insights I got during fasting. I had taken notes and once in a while I looked over them with amazement.*

*A few months later my body had put on weight again.*

*I decided to fast once a week.*

*Initially I sensed headaches and circulatory disturbances. These kinds of symptoms, however, disappeared quite quickly. I probably had already detoxified a bit.*

*I still do a fast once a week for 24 hours. I really like it to be a weekly event. It relaxes me. I get to rest. My pulse beats more slowly, my breathing becomes deeper;*

*I have a lot of time and ponder less.*
*I also feel more light-hearted and my muscles loosen up. I am less tense.*
*Once a year I do a longer fast. It's usually less than five days in a row, which is sufficient for my weight.*
*I can tolerate a longer fast much better now.*
*Each time I get lavished with more clarity and insights.*
*I feel the essence inside of me and also around me.*
*I realize moderate exercising is the most important key factor while fasting. It helps to get rid of toxins, keeps the circulation going and leads to well-being.*

Inner cleansing is just a technique. It is applied because of the unnatural lifestyle we are living.

It is not in creation's natural flow.

Due to actual discrepancies it is a very helpful tool. The feeling of being 'empty' and then to be filled with the all present life energy is such an amazing experience.

When you're void, this 'force' finally gets space to unfold and express itself within you.

It is a really good technique for cleansing and detoxifying.

It might not be necessary for very healthy and conscious people.

Sick people, however, should definitely give it a try.

# 6. Excursus: Wild plants in practice

From now on, wild plants might be part of your diet. The question is how to approach the whole thing?

At first, observe your natural environment for a while. Go for walks in nature or even in town and take a closer look at plant life around you.

Even while doing every-day errands you can see many common plants. You'll get familiar with them in a very relaxed and natural way just by giving them attention, by observing their presence wherever you are. You will eventually notice certain plants quite frequently. You may see them all over. Gradually, you start memorizing flora around you in an automatic way.

That's a good base to go into detail. You can now start to identify edible plants by reading books on this topic or by attending a class.

It won't take long until you know where to find something to nibble.

Stop believing that rare things, being hard to get and having the highest prices, will help you most.

It is not the plant from the deepest jungle; it is not that rare herb only a few people have access to that will be your salvation.

Be attentive.

Be aware, often-times people are particularly interested in only your money.

Life, however, is simple and easy. Mostly it's the plant in your immediate area, often times so-called 'weeds', that nourish you best. The whole thing is not complicated at all, but instead it feels quite pleasant. Shouldn't life be this way?

It's nice to observe an increase of interest in edible wild plants. Integrating a small vegetable garden in everyday life is becoming more common. A generally high demand for regional organic products can be noticed.

With time, you'll be more receptive to the world of plants. You'll develop a special sense and find your own approach to surrounding flora.

Too often we're just carelessly passing by.

Taking a closer look, you will notice a plant is a very graceful being. It doesn't complain. It withstands all weather conditions. It 'is' and follows the tasks it is assigned. It is patient and acts in an intelligent way. It decides to take rest in winter. In spring its leaves and flowers grow. It patiently waits until seeds and fruits ripen. It provides habitat. It gives us food and, above all, it produces our life's base: Oxygen to breathe.

At first, memorize the most poisonous plants of your area.

Poisonous plants exist because you're not the universe's centre and other organisms might benefit from them.

If you're in doubt about a plant's edibility, just skip it for this time. Instead eat plants you know. You can always get more information later by identifying a special plant, doing research on its edible or poisonous qualities.

Always eat from a variety of different plants. Never consume a single wild plant in excess.

Just take a little bit from each different plant. Never eat consistently on only one plant over a long period of time.

If you come across a plant you don't have any knowledge about, take a close look before you touch it. There can always be small spines or thorns somewhere. You might also encounter bees hiding in edible flowers, so be a little bit careful.

You have many senses, why not use them? There is a reason why you're equipped with all these organs.

Take a plant's leaf you're interested in and grind it between your fingers. As a result there might be a scent to perceive. If the odour is extremely unpleasant, this plant is probably not meant for you.

Keep in mind that flowers with a nice fragrance aren't automatically safe to eat. In fact, some of the most beautiful and fragrant flowering plants are highly toxic.

If you're just starting, it's necessary to gather information about your surrounding flora.

You might also want to check the environment of the plants you intend to eat.

Do they grow in a park or garden regularly treated with insecticides?

Farmer's fields and surrounding areas are also sprayed quite often.

Take caution while handling plants and flowers from commercial dealers. Don't eat roses your husband bought for your anniversary.

Try to avoid plants that are exposed to lots of traffic.

Of course, it's wonderful to have your own garden. Remember though to eat from different places with different soil. Your system wants to be provided with a variety of nutrients and micro-organisms.

This depends on soil and environmental exposure. Soil is not composed the same way wherever you go. Environmental impacts differ too. Considering our original program, we are probably not made to be sedentary, obtaining food from only one type of soil.

Honour the plant you're eating and show it some respect. Remove only as many parts as necessary. Don't kill it by pulling out entire root systems or taking away all its foliage and flowers. Do your foraging from a variety of plants, so that in the future you will also have something to eat.

Fortunately, there are already quite a few books available on edible wild plants. While studying, or in case someone else is teaching you, keep those plants in mind which you can eat in a raw state. Information given on edible plants generally doesn't exclude cooking processes. In common literature, raw edible plants are most often referred as to be "good herbs for salads". Indeed, there are a wide variety of wild plants that are toxic when eaten raw. Those plants can only be consumed after being processed. Knowing this detail you have to be vigilant. Always make sure to check a plant's edibility in a raw state.

Each climate has different vegetation patterns. I had to realize that when travelling to other climate zones. Getting to know the world's flora is a never-ending story. Plant life on this planet is incredibly large and diverse: plants of deep tropical areas, plants of cooler mountain regions or those in front of our doorsteps.

The first arrival in a different climate zone brought me down to Earth. I looked around and didn't recognize a single plant.

What was I supposed to do now?

What would I eat?

I used the 'procedure' mentioned earlier.

At first, I decided to consciously observe my natural environment. For a certain time I simply watched plants around me. I was noticing their presence while passing by. I automatically memorized common flora, because I always got to see the same type of plants over and over again. After a while I got clearer about typical vegetation patterns. I started to read books on the flora of the country in which I was living. If this wasn't possible, I turned to books on a nearby countries' flora with a similar climate.

I always made sure to memorize the most poisonous plants of the area. Then I started to find out more about the flora I was surrounded with. After identifying some common plants, I did some research on potential toxic properties. I also looked for information about possible humans already using this kind of plant as a resource. I asked local people for advice. I had to learn that not all information given to me turned out to be true.

Often-times, when people recommended a certain type of plant as safe to eat in a raw state, it ended up being edible only when cooked.

Sometimes it's better to take some caution when adopting other people's advice.

Check important information by yourself, especially if you have any doubts.

Look carefully before you touch something. You're not the only creature on planet Earth. A plant's world provides habitat for many organisms.

Unfortunately, we have lost most knowledge about edible plants.

If you're not sure about a plant's edibility, smell it first. Then ingest only a tiny bit. Wait a few hours and see if your system tolerates it. If you feel quite well, you might try a bit more next time.

Remember to take just a little bit of lesser known plants. Always eat more from a variety. Never feed on one type of plant only.


Illustrating all kinds of edible plants would go beyond this book's scope. Plenty of literature is already available. To name some examples for temperate climate zones: dandelion, ground elder (Aegopodium podagraria), rose petals or young leaves of a linden tree (Tilia) can be quite a treat. In a more 'Mediterranean' climate defined by hot, dry summers and temperate, wet winters, I'd recommend wild fennel (Foeniculum vulgare), fruits of the western strawberry tree (Arbutus unedo), blackberry leaves and consumption of wild figs. In tropical areas plenty of fresh young coconuts are waiting for you. You can also eat different kinds of hibiscus plants, leaves of costus and flowers of Jamaica vervain (Stachytarpheta jamaicensis).

Enjoy your meal.

# 7. And now?

Our body is like the universe. It is very complex. Instead of putting too much focus on details, it should therefore be comprehended in a holistic way. Most health problems in modern society can't be solved by a quick, temporary fix in one specific body part. For chronically ill people to reach a state of well-being, it is indispensable to take a holistic approach on our interwoven system.

What is the best medicine?

We need to rethink and no longer talk about 'medicine'.

Instead of trying to find cures, it's about prevention from diseases through a healthy and species appropriate lifestyle. It seems to be the best solution for society's health problems.


Stick to a healthy lifestyle so that you don't get sick in the first place.

These days you're already preparing the base to prevent getting seriously ill later in your life.

When time arrives, your body may die naturally, free of suffering and looking back on a beautiful life. Life force, which was flowing through your system, will naturally find an ending. It will peacefully disappear from your body. Until then, enjoy your life in a healthy way. It has so much to offer, maybe more than you can ever imagine.

Relax and be prepared. Things you previously put a lot of value on might be put into perspective. They might change.

You realize life is flow: It is a coming and going, a dying and renewing. Everything is in unison, following a set rhythm. You feel held by creation, always prepared to let go.

At the beginning I mentioned diseases I had. Before discovering and consciously choosing a natural, healthy lifestyle, I had taken more than 10,000 individual prescription pills over a period of several years. Looking back on my former health state, I find it quite shocking.

What is my system supposed to do with all this stuff? Ultimately, I can only report from my own experiences.

Applying a species appropriate lifestyle, in the first year I managed to take 40 pills a year instead of 1000. In the second year, I only needed five pills. In the third year I didn't have to take any kind of medicine. This hasn't changed so far.

Reading about my experiences should be enough now.

Your conscious mind might be encouraged.

If this is the case, just begin putting things into practice.

There is a beautiful old folk saying: "There is nothing good, unless you do it".

Take heart.

Just do it and see what happens.

What do you have to lose?

Until you have tried it yourself, try not to over-criticize this whole approach. Who knows? Despite all scepticism, maybe there is some truth to be found.

*I was sitting on a meadow when all of the sudden my view started to change. It felt like I had been wearing an opaque veil on my eyes. Suddenly I felt this veil being removed. It opened up like a curtain and I perceived my environment differently. Colours around me were brighter, richer and more lucid. The green of the grass and the blue of the sky were beaming and gleaming in rich, full tones.*

*I was flabbergasted. I had never seen my environment like this.*

*I started to understand what was going on and I was just amazed by the beauty I was surrounded with.*

# Epilogue

There will never be a perfect teaching, nor an immaculate theory made up by human beings.

If you get in touch with new ideas, never get stuck in doubts because of small details and discard everything new you just experienced. You will always find something that doesn't suit you, something that isn't perfect. Never mind that. Look at the big picture. Look at the essence and try to 'feel' if you can find truth for yourself.

Stop arguing about minor things: Life is short.

Let go of constant reasoning and the need of being right all the time. Quit this way of thinking, but instead consciously strive for harmony and unity.

Often-times, teachers can firmly hold on to their one-sided points of view. They can be very caught up in their efforts to be right. For years they unnecessarily debate and argue on small details. Closing their minds, they cut themselves off from a greater vision, from integration.

That's a waste of valuable life energy.

Why do we work against each other?

Instead, let's work together.

We should really quit the habit of debating on small details.

Instead, let us use our time for better and more beautiful things.

It's about a larger, an all-encompassing principle: connecting with the ever-present life energy, meaning love. We therefore shouldn't fight or insist, but try to pull together in order to create more awareness, peace and health. Let's find access to our true nature, to its inherent potential.

It's not about living like a savage; it's about behaving more appropriately to our species, about being human for real.

I think this is just a first step, helping us to be back in conjunction with creation. From here, we will be guided on further paths, paths that are still unknown to us.

By re-accessing creation's forces we might start to 'think', 'feel' and 'act' in ways that differ from present patterns, ways that currently seem to be out of reach.

Let us therefore be curious.

Let us stay open for leaps of awareness that are likely to reach us in our near future.

I believe in it.

*Ludwig Anderson,*
*written in October 2013*

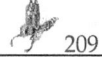

# Literature

Konz, Franz: *Der grosse Gesundheits-Konz.* Universitas, 2001 (available only in german language)

Byrne, Rhonda: *The Secret.* 2007. Atria Books/Beyond Words, 2006.

Castenada, Carlos: *Various books.*

Chopra, Deepak: *The Book of Secrets.* Three Rivers Press, 2005.

Hay, Louis: *You can heal your life.* Hay House, 1984.

Kabat-Zinn, Jon: *Mindfulness for Beginners.* Sounds True, 2011.

Martin, Franklin et al.: *Edible Leaves of the Tropics.* Echo, 1998.

McDougall, Christopher: *Born to run.* Knopf, 2010.

Merrill, Elmer D.: *Emergency food plants and poisonous plants of the islands of the pacific.* United States War Dept.., 1923.

Schatalova, Galina: *Wir fressen uns zu Tode*. Goldmann Verlag, 2002 (available only in german and russian language).

Thoreau, Henry D.: *Walden*. Various publishers. Original edition 1854.

Rothkranz, Markus: *Heal Yourself 101*. Rothkranz Publishing, 2011.

Ruiz, Don Miguel: *The Four Agreements*. Amber-Allen, 2004.

Walsch, Neale D.: *Conversations with God*. G. P. Putnam's Sons, 1996.

Zuchowski, Willow: *Tropical plants of Costa Rica: A guide to native flora and exotic flora*. Zona Tropical, 2007.

Database 'Plants for a Future': www.pfaf.org

Copyright © Ludwig Anderson 2013
**ludwig.anderson@outlook.com**

Naturally I am healthy/Ludwig Anderson

ISBN-13: 978-1500766542
Published by Stefanie Nicole Gogol, Lechenicherstr. 16
50937 Köln

Printed by Amazon Distribution Gmbh

www.ingramcontent.com/pod-product-compliance
Lightning Source LLC
Chambersburg PA
CBHW070108290526
45789CB00005B/1966